Flow Diagrams in Advanced Cancer and Other Diseases

Flow Diagrams in
Advanced Cancer and Other Diseases

Edited by

Claud Regnard

St Oswald's Hospice, Newcastle-upon-Tyne

and

Jo Hockley

Western General Hospitals NHS Trust, Edinburgh

Foreword by
Derek Doyle

Edward Arnold
A member of the Hodder Headline Group
LONDON   BOSTON   MELBOURNE   AUCKLAND

First published in Great Britain in 1995 by
Edward Arnold, a division of Hodder Headline PLC,
338 Euston Road, London NW1 3BH

British Library Cataloguing in Publication Data
A catalogue record for this book is available from the British Library

ISBN 0 340 61389 0

1 2 3 4 5   95 96 97 98 99

Typeset in Caslon by GreenGate Publishing Services, Tonbridge, Kent
Printed and bound in Great Britain by the Bath Press, Bath, Avon

Contents

Foreword

Times have certainly changed! I remember, when taking up my present post in the 1970s, being told by an elderly, retired and distinguished physician that it had taken him fully three days to learn how to care for the dying. 'Morphine is a wonderful drug, but it takes a few days to learn how to use it!' Since then we have all been inspired by the hospice movement and learned that it is never true to say, 'There is nothing more we can do', because there is always something we can offer, whether it is palliation of physical or emotional problems, a sensitive ear for spiritual issues, or our communication skills to help the patient and family. Terminal care has developed into palliative care, now both a medical and nursing speciality, focusing not on death but on quality of living, harnessing the skills of physicians, nurses and many paramedical colleagues, and demanding from all the highest professional skills and generous sharing of our humanity.

This recognition of the kaleidoscope of suffering amenable to palliation has had its implications. One is an educated understanding of disease processes and the suffering each stage may bring. This is not easy because doctors have, for too long, regarded symptoms merely as diagnostic indicators, rather than the reflections of a patient's suffering and loss, where each new symptom calls for the doctor to provide identification, evaluation, explanation and relief, whilst never losing sight that the underlying pathology will continue its relentless course. Another implication is that professional carers must learn a new therapeutic discipline, its goal being the relief of suffering rather than the eradication of a pathology. Standard drugs may now have to be employed in different ways, demanding of the prescriber a detailed knowledge of each, in situations where polypharmacy may be the norm. Each drug must be used to advantage without in any way adding to the burdens already borne by the patient. Such clinical care is not simple and may often be very complex, requiring an inter-professional, rather than multi-professional approach, where each professional group can scarcely function or continue without the others.

The need for good research and dissemination of evaluated palliation regimens was one reason for our establishing the journal *Palliative Medicine*, now the foremost journal on the subject worldwide. A feature of the journal has been its flow diagrams, clearly appreciated and found useful because they are reproduced or alluded to in many other reference works, and are now brought together in this volume. Their importance and usefulness can hardly be exaggerated. They emphasise a systematic and logical approach. They challenge clinical skills and assume a sound and comprehensive knowledge of pharmacology. They remind us that each symptom, each facet of suffering, is important and demands our attention. They remind us, if indeed we still need such a reminder, that there is always something we can do! Putting their principles into practice will take more than a few days, but our patients deserve the best and these flow diagrams will help us to offer it.

Derek Doyle
Consultant in Palliative Medicine
First Editor in Chief, *Palliative Medicine*
St. Columba's Hospice,
Edinburgh, UK
1995

Contributors

Sam Ahmedzai

Professor of Palliative Medicine, Section of Palliative Medicine, Royal Hallamshire Hospital, and University of Sheffield, Sheffield, UK.

Caroline Badger

Macmillan Nurse Consultant in Lymphoedema

Sue Bale

Director of Nursing Research, Wound Healing Research Unit, University Department of Surgery, Unversity of Wales College of Medicine, Cardiff, UK.

Mary Comiskey

Senior Registrar in Palliative Medicine, St. Oswald's Hospice, Newcastle-upon-Tyne, UK.

Derek Doyle

Medical Director and Consultant in Palliative Medicine, St. Columba's Hospice; member of Clinical Teaching staff, Department of Medicine, University of Edinburgh, Edinburgh, UK.

Ann Faulkner

Professor of Communication in Health Care, University of Sheffield Medical School; Deputy Director, Trent Palliative Care Centre, Sheffield, UK.

Sarah Fitton

Ward Sister, St. Oswald's Hospice, Newcastle-upon-Tyne, UK.

Jo Hockley

Clinical Nurse Specialist in Palliative Care, Western General Hospitals Trust, Edinburgh, UK.

Peter Maguire

Honorary Consultant Psychiatrist; Director of Cancer Research Campaign; Psychological Medicine Group, Christie Hospital, Manchester, UK.

Wendy Makin

Consultant in Palliative Medicine, St. Oswald's Hospice; Honorary Consultant Clinical Oncologist, Northern Centre for Cancer Treatment; Newcastle-upon-Tyne, UK.

Kathryn Mannix

Senior Registrar in Palliative Medicine, St. Oswald's Hospice, Newcastle-upon-Tyne, UK.

Claud Regnard

Medical Director, St. Oswald's Hospice; Honorary Consultant in Palliative Medicine, Royal Victoria Infirmary; Honorary Lecturer in Pharmacological Sciences, University of Newcastle-upon-Tyne; UK.

Jackie Saunders

Clinical Nurse Specialist – Palliative Care, West Suffolk Hospital, Bury St Edmunds, UK.

Nick Smith

Staff Therapist and Trainer, Institute of Family Therapy, London, UK.

Averil Stedeford

Former Consultant in Psychological Medicine, Sir Michael Sobell House, Oxford, UK.

John W Thompson

Honorary Physician and Honorary Consultant in Medical Studies, St. Oswald's Hospice; Emeritus Professor of Pharmacology, University of Newcastle-upon-Tyne; Emeritus Consultant Clinical Pharmacologist, Newcastle Health Authority; Former Director, Pain Relief Clinic, Royal Victoria Infirmary, Newcastle-upon-Tyne; UK

Preface

Effective palliative care requires clear decisions to be made in the face of complex issues, with an interdisciplinary approach that values different skills and expertise. However, the clarity of decisions, can be clouded by an unfamiliar problem, incomplete understanding, and the strength of emotions involved. The consequence is that a sensible, logical and intelligent carer will make decisions that seem correct at the time, but turn out to be wholly inappropriate. In malignancy, Robert Twycross has called this a 'cancer fog', but it could equally be a 'motor neurone disease fog', or an 'AIDS fog'. None of us is immune from its effects, but knowing where the key decisions lie makes a path through the fog possible. First published in the journal, *Palliative Medicine*, these flow diagrams have all been revised and updated. They suggest which are the key clinical decisions, and show a logical path through the problems. We hope that these diagrams will clarify the issues for carers and make successful management more likely.

Claud Regnard

Jo Hockley

1995

Using the flow diagrams

These flow diagrams were designed to follow a reading pattern where each part of the diagram reads from left to right. This usually leads you to the next line (in the same way as text), but occasionally you are returned to the same line, implying a particular condition must be met before you can move on. Key clinical decisions are in shaded boxes. For nearly all the clinical decisions in the diagrams, affirmative answers read horizontally, while negative answers lead you to the next line of the diagram. These answers lead you to action boxes (treatments or decisions), and each action is marked with a ● bullet point. Each flow of decisions will lead you through most or all of the key decisions, and the diagrams usually return you to the beginning, forming a decision loop that implies repeated assessments. The accompanying notes to each flow diagram explain and expand the issues covered. We hope these design points not only make it easier to read, but also make it easier to remember the clinical decisions for each problem.

Acknowledgements

We are grateful to the authors for their close collaboration in each flow diagram, and we are indebted to Derek Doyle for his support and encouragement. Our thanks also go to David Mackin and Jenny McQueen who patiently redesigned the flow diagrams, and to many colleagues who advised us.

1 Eliciting the Current Problems

Peter Maguire
Ann Faulkner
Claud Regnard

The assessment of a patient, relative or partner is an integral part of clinical management. It should be conducted in a way that maximises the opportunity of the individual disclosing all their main problems, whether physical, social or psychological in nature. Unfortunately, professional carers can be uncertain of their ability to do this. This flow diagram leads the carer through key points in the assessment interview.

The importance of being able to elicit psychosocial as well as physical problems is only slowly gaining a place in general professional training. Consequently some professional carers lack confidence in their ability to do this at all, or to do it without taking too much time. This flow diagram indicates the key decisions that need to be made, and the strategies to be used if an assessment interview is to be of optimal use to both the individual and the professional carer.

Setting the scene

Seeing the person alone is preferable. People often deliberately withhold important information if they are first seen with a partner, relative or friend. The individual may wish to protect their companion from the reality of their prognosis, suffering and fears, or may not usually confide problems to that person. Sometimes the companion may 'talk over' the anxious individual.

When time is short establish which problem the person most wants help with. Try to elicit its nature and severity, and how the person perceives and feels about the problem. Explain the action to be taken and that you will attend to any other problems later.

Time limits should be negotiated. When this is done (and adhered to), people disclose their problems more quickly and feel safer. It also minimises the risk of dependency.

Taking notes will avoid your forgetting important cues about possible problem areas and will enable you to clarify those areas adequately. Noting down key data tells the person you are taking their problems seriously. It does *not* hinder disclosure.

Sharing information with the team is important. Proper care of patients requires a team of people from different disciplines who have complementary skills. Pooling of information about the patient and the family maximises that care. It also minimises the risk of dependency, unrealistic expectations and professional over involvement.

Main strategy

Eliciting problems is easier if the professional carer does not interrupt the person in the middle of speaking. Summarising the problems makes it clear you have been listening and enables you to check if the list is correct.

Exploring each problem is necessary to understand it fully, and to see how the person perceives it and has reacted to it.

Distress: Most distressed patients or relatives want you to acknowledge their distress and help them explain how distressed they are and why. Even if you cannot resolve all their problems, they will feel better for 'off-loading' them. You will only risk causing harm if you insist on individuals talking about a problem that they have stated is too painful to discuss. So always check that they can bear to talk about it.

Concluding within your agreed time prevents you being drawn into further discussion. Otherwise the person may believe they have unlimited time, may become more demanding and prevent you from spending sufficient time with your other patients, relatives and partners.

SET THE SCENE
Greet person and introduce yourself by name and status.

IS THE PERSON ACCOMPANIED? — YES →
- If space or room is available, explain you prefer to see person on their own first.
- **If person agrees:** arrange to see them alone.
- **If person disagrees:** see them with an accompanying person.

NO ↓

- If time too short or patient too unwell for a full interview of 30 minutes: Focus on recent change point, or elicit major problems only

- Explain your role and objectives.
DOES PERSON OBJECT TO YOUR ROLE AND/OR OBJECTIVES? — YES →
- Explore the reasons
- **If person refuses further negotiation:** no further action.
- **If person agrees:** renegotiate objectives, e.g. concentrate on main problem only.

NO ↓

- Mention time available for interview.
DOES PERSON OBJECT TO TIME AVAILABLE? — YES →
- **If time is too short:** Explore the reasons and attempt to negotiate follow up interviews:
  - person objects to negotiation: acknowledge this and end interview.
  - person agrees to negotiation: arrange further, longer interview and (with person's agreement) try and get as far as possible today.
- **If time is too long:** Explore reasons and negotiate more limited objectives, e.g. main problem only.

NO ↓

- Mention that you would like to take notes during interview.
DOES PERSON OBJECT TO YOU TAKING NOTES? — YES →
- Explore the reasons
- **If person objects to negotiation:** agree that notes will not be taken.
- **If person agrees to negotiation:** take notes of what has been agreed (e.g. person may wish certain data to be left unrecorded).

NO ↓

- Mention that you are the member of a team and need to be able to share what is discussed with colleagues.
DOES PERSON OBJECT TO SHARING INFORMATION WITH THE TEAM? — YES →
Person insists that certain information is kept secret:
- Advise person not to tell you that since you cannot agree to secrecy.
- **If person objects:** offer to refer to a professionally supported counsellor.
- **If person agrees:** go to main strategy.

NO ↓

Person accepts need to share.

↓

GO TO MAIN STRATEGY

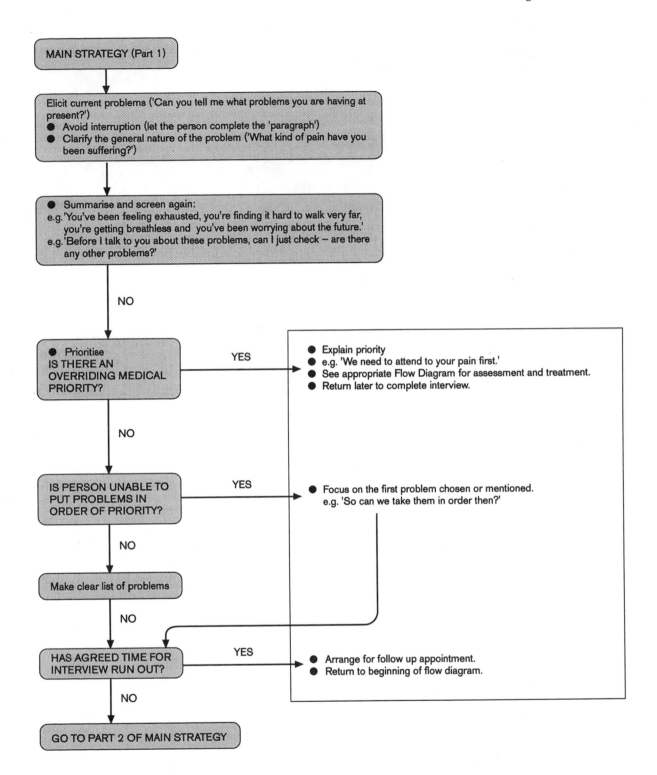

MAIN STRATEGY (Part 1)

Elicit current problems ('Can you tell me what problems you are having at present?')
● Avoid interruption (let the person complete the 'paragraph')
● Clarify the general nature of the problem ('What kind of pain have you been suffering?')

● Summarise and screen again:
e.g. 'You've been feeling exhausted, you're finding it hard to walk very far, you're getting breathless and you've been worrying about the future.'
e.g. 'Before I talk to you about these problems, can I just check — are there any other problems?'

NO

● Prioritise
IS THERE AN OVERRIDING MEDICAL PRIORITY?

YES

● Explain priority
● e.g. 'We need to attend to your pain first.'
● See appropriate Flow Diagram for assessment and treatment.
● Return later to complete interview.

NO

IS PERSON UNABLE TO PUT PROBLEMS IN ORDER OF PRIORITY?

YES

● Focus on the first problem chosen or mentioned.
e.g. 'So can we take them in order then?'

NO

Make clear list of problems

NO

HAS AGREED TIME FOR INTERVIEW RUN OUT?

YES

● Arrange for follow up appointment.
● Return to beginning of flow diagram.

NO

GO TO PART 2 OF MAIN STRATEGY

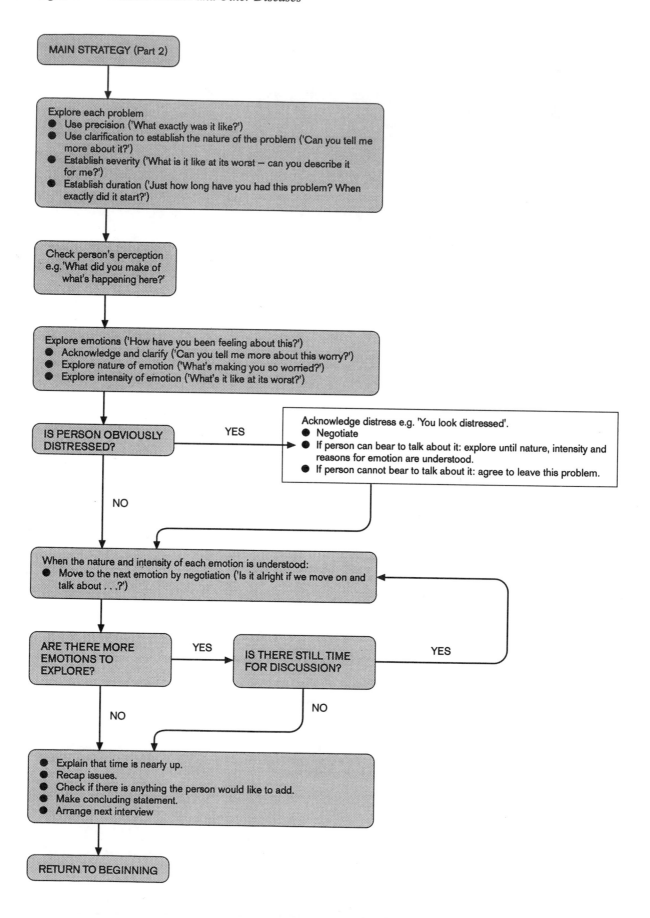

2 Pain

John W Thompson
Claud Regnard

The complex nature of pain should not deflect the carer from the need to assess the precipitating cause of each pain. This flow diagram describes the clinical decisions required in assessing pain, suggests likely causes and outlines treatment.

Introduction

Pain is a complex physiological and emotional experience which may make its management appear a daunting task. This difficulty can be lessened, however, if the approach is sensitive and methodical. Successful management is more likely if the cornerstones of assessment (including diagnosis), planning (including goal setting), treatment and reassessment are followed for each pain, with each step involving the patient. This flow diagram demonstrates the clinical decisions required in assessment, suggests likely diagnoses for each category, and briefly outlines the treatment for each cause of pain.

Terminology

There is still confusion and disagreement on pain terminology, and as far as possible a clinically based terminology has been used for this flow diagram.

Initial approach

The care taken over managing pain is a clear demonstration to the patient that the carer believes the patient is distressed by their pain. Pain severity is difficult to assess and it is better to rely on the extent to which the pain is limiting the patient's daily activities. It is worthwhile eliciting the patient's goals, since if these prove to be inappropriate, the patient will need help in understanding and accepting this conflict. Simple measures, such as correct positioning, and ensuring basic needs are prerequisites to a successful approach.

Pain related to movement

This implies pain precipitated or worsened by movement.

Pain on the slightest passive movement induced by the examiner suggests a fracture, but is occasionally seen with nerve compression and soft tissue inflammation due to tumour or infection. Such pain may be severe and prevent even basic patient care. The immediate priority is to relieve distress at rest – immobilisation can be sufficient, but a strong opioid or even titrated sedation (e.g. midazolam by subcutaneous infusion[1]), may be required. Spinal analgesia can be invaluable in such situations,[2,3] and allow time to plan further action, such as elective orthopaedic surgery.

Pain elicited during examination when a bone is stressed (e.g. by application of pressure to a femoral shaft, or by percussion over vertebrae) may be due to an underlying bone metastasis with cortical destruction. The resulting skeletal instability is unlikely to respond well to strong opioids or to nonsteroidal antiinflammatory drugs (NSAIDs), until the instability is resolved by surgery, by treating the metastasis (usually with radiotherapy) or by encouraging bone healing (e.g. bisphosphonates in breast carcinoma).[4] Patients with pain at rest from bone metastases can be helped with a strong opioid. A small proportion of such patients may also be helped by NSAIDs, although there is no clear evidence that the majority of patients with bone metastatic pain benefit from these drugs. If the pain elicited on examination radiates along the distribution of a discrete nerve, this suggests accompanying nerve compression, which may require regional anaesthesia, or high dose dexamethasone.

Pain elicited by asking the patient to make a movement against resistance may also be due to a bone abnormality, but often arises from within skeletal muscle. The presence of a discretely tender spot, often with an underlying band of muscle in spasm, is typical of a myofascial trigger point. Such pains have typical sites and radiations depending on the muscle involved,[5] and respond to local treatment of the trigger point with local anaesthesia, transcutaneous electrical nerve stimulation (TENS),[6] or dry needling. Skeletal muscle strain and spasm may also respond to heat and massage, although spasm occasionally requires a systemic antispastic such as baclofen.

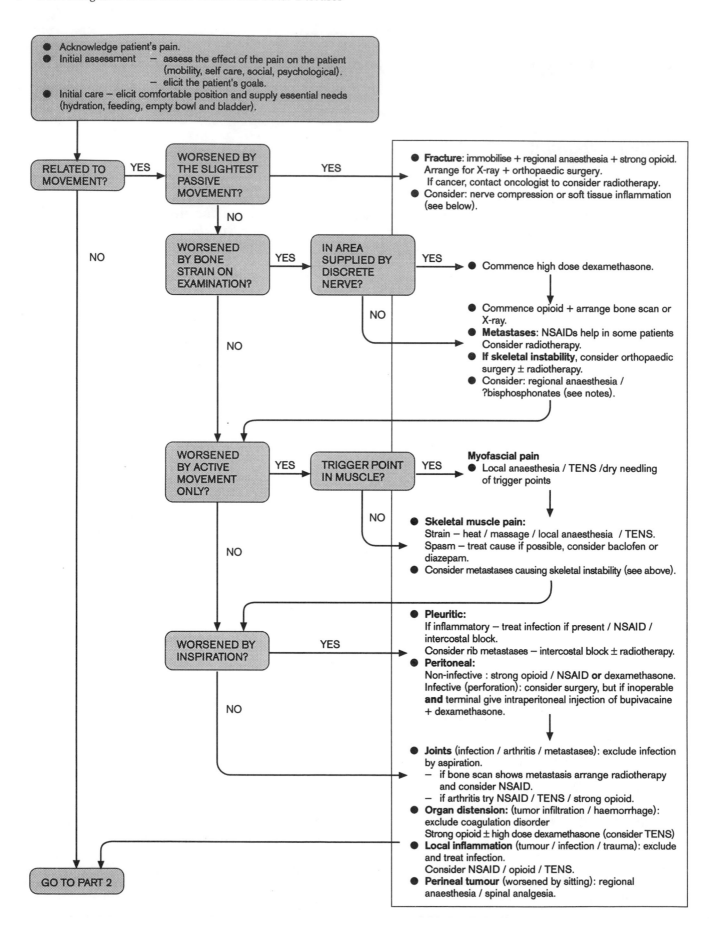

Pain worsened by inspiration may be due to problems arising within the chest wall and these require specific treatments. Peritoneal inflammation can be caused by peritoneal metastases which may respond to a strong opioid +/– NSAID.

Other movement-related pains may arise from joints, organ distension (e.g. hepatomegaly) or local inflammation, and the management will depend on the cause.

Periodic pain

Regular, sharp episodes of pain, suggest smooth muscle spasm (colic), with the site and radiation depending on the source. Occasionally such a spasm is continuous, giving a steady pain lasting 10–30 minutes, but the site, radiation and treatment are the same. Treatment involves either removing the source of irritation (e.g. drugs irritating the bowel), instillations of topical local anaesthesia (in bladder irritation due to tumour), or the use of an antispasmodic (e.g. hyoscine butylbromide).

Pain related to eating

This may be due to problems with swallowing, or with the mouth, oesophagus or stomach. Treatment will depend on the cause (see also the flow diagram on *Mouth Care*).

Pain with associated skin damage or disease

Specific skin problems will require appropriate treatment.

Unpleasant sensory changes at rest

This type of pain is usually due to nerve damage, and does not involve pain receptors. This neuropathic pain can be due to continuing nerve damage (neuralgia), or can persist after the damage has occurred (deafferentation pain, sympathetically maintained pain). Following damage to a nerve pathway (often a peripheral nerve or root), neuropathic pain can occur within 1–3 months, occasionally in hours. Most neuropathic pains have a dermatomal or peripheral nerve distribution, but a few have a vascular distribution due to altered sympathetic activity, and these are usually accompanied by skin changes due to sympathetic hyperactivity in the initial stages, followed later by hypoactivity. Neuropathic pains are described with words such as burning, shooting, pins and needles, sandpaper, scalding, freezing. Altered sensation is an important sign, particularly hyperaesthesia (increased sensitivity to stroking) or allodynia (pain that is provoked by a normally non-painful stimulus such as stroking).

In managing neuropathic pain, reversible causes of painful neuropathy such as B12 deficiency need to be excluded. Although neuropathic pain is usually partly or totally unresponsive to opioids, in some conditions such as cancer it is often part of a mixed pain and it is worth starting a trial with morphine since other components of the pain may respond. Otherwise, low doses of tricyclic antidepressants, or anticonvulsants in standard doses, can be effective singly or in combination. In sympathetic dependent pain, that associated with sympathetic hyperactive pain can be helped by a chemical sympathectomy, while the application of a TENS over the supplying artery can occasionally help pain associated with sympathetic hypoactivity. Other drugs and techniques can be useful, and the advice of a pain specialist is essential if the first line treatments are ineffective.

Pain in an area supplied by a peripheral nerve

Compression of a nerve root, plexus or peripheral nerve may respond to a strong opioid with or without high dose dexamethasone. Inflammation may be helped by a nonsteroidal antiinflammatory drug.

Signs and symptoms suggesting a CNS lesion

Cord compression needs to be assessed and treated urgently – treatment can be worthwhile even in a patient with a prognosis of a few weeks. Cranial nerve pain (trigeminal, vagal or glossopharyngeal) may respond to a strong opioid with or without dexamethasone; and unpleasant sensory changes at rest suggest a neuropathic pain which needs specific treatment (see above). Pain due to thalamic metastases may respond to dexamethasone with or without cranial irradiation, or to a amitriptyline/distigmine combination.[8] Meningeal pain due to metastases may also require strong opioids with or without dexamethasone.

If the cause of pain is still undecided

If the cause of pain is still undecided consider arterial insufficiency, infection and malignant infiltration of bone or soft tissue. Occasionally some pains present in an atypical way. For example, neuropathic pain may present without sensory changes, and is only suspected when it responds to one of the treatments for neuropathic pain.

Explanation and goal setting

Once the likely cause of pain has been elicited, it follows that the likely treatment is known and it becomes possible to explain this to the patient – it is often a relief to patients that a likely cause (and therefore treatment) is now known. Realistic goals then need to be set. These goals need to be negotiated with the patient – for example, expecting freedom from pain on walking in the presence of skeletal instability will result in disappointment for patient and carers alike.

If the pain is still present

If despite a careful assessment and appropriate treatment, the pain is still present then it is worth considering unresolved psychosocial issues, poor compliance with medication, or inappropriate analgesic dose or timing. Since new pains can arise in the site of the original pain, persistent pain should prompt reassessment as described in the flow diagram.

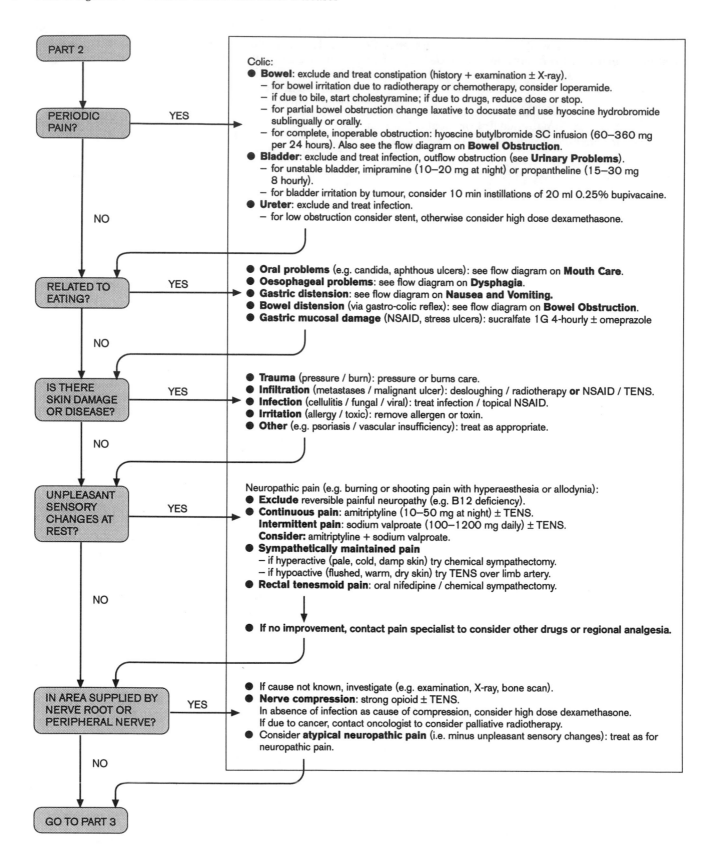

PART 2

PERIODIC PAIN? — YES →

Colic:
- **Bowel**: exclude and treat constipation (history + examination ± X-ray).
  - for bowel irritation due to radiotherapy or chemotherapy, consider loperamide.
  - if due to bile, start cholestyramine; if due to drugs, reduce dose or stop.
  - for partial bowel obstruction change laxative to docusate and use hyoscine hydrobromide sublingually or orally.
  - for complete, inoperable obstruction: hyoscine butylbromide SC infusion (60–360 mg per 24 hours). Also see the flow diagram on **Bowel Obstruction**.
- **Bladder**: exclude and treat infection, outflow obstruction (see **Urinary Problems**).
  - for unstable bladder, imipramine (10–20 mg at night) or propantheline (15–30 mg 8 hourly).
  - for bladder irritation by tumour, consider 10 min instillations of 20 ml 0.25% bupivacaine.
- **Ureter**: exclude and treat infection.
  - for low obstruction consider stent, otherwise consider high dose dexamethasone.

NO ↓

RELATED TO EATING? — YES →

- **Oral problems** (e.g. candida, aphthous ulcers): see flow diagram on **Mouth Care**.
- **Oesophageal problems**: see flow diagram on **Dysphagia**.
- **Gastric distension**: see flow diagram on **Nausea and Vomiting.**
- **Bowel distension** (via gastro-colic reflex): see flow diagram on **Bowel Obstruction**.
- **Gastric mucosal damage** (NSAID, stress ulcers): sucralfate 1G 4-hourly ± omeprazole

NO ↓

IS THERE SKIN DAMAGE OR DISEASE? — YES →

- **Trauma** (pressure / burn): pressure or burns care.
- **Infiltration** (metastases / malignant ulcer): desloughing / radiotherapy **or** NSAID / TENS.
- **Infection** (cellulitis / fungal / viral): treat infection / topical NSAID.
- **Irritation** (allergy / toxic): remove allergen or toxin.
- **Other** (e.g. psoriasis / vascular insufficiency): treat as appropriate.

NO ↓

UNPLEASANT SENSORY CHANGES AT REST? — YES →

Neuropathic pain (e.g. burning or shooting pain with hyperaesthesia or allodynia):
- **Exclude** reversible painful neuropathy (e.g. B12 deficiency).
- **Continuous pain**: amitriptyline (10–50 mg at night) ± TENS.
  Intermittent pain: sodium valproate (100–1200 mg daily) ± TENS.
  Consider: amitriptyline + sodium valproate.
- **Sympathetically maintained pain**
  - if hyperactive (pale, cold, damp skin) try chemical sympathectomy.
  - if hypoactive (flushed, warm, dry skin) try TENS over limb artery.
- **Rectal tenesmoid pain**: oral nifedipine / chemical sympathectomy.

- If no improvement, contact pain specialist to consider other drugs or regional analgesia.

NO ↓

IN AREA SUPPLIED BY NERVE ROOT OR PERIPHERAL NERVE? — YES →

- If cause not known, investigate (e.g. examination, X-ray, bone scan).
- **Nerve compression**: strong opioid ± TENS.
  In absence of infection as cause of compression, consider high dose dexamethasone.
  If due to cancer, contact oncologist to consider palliative radiotherapy.
- Consider **atypical neuropathic pain** (i.e. minus unpleasant sensory changes): treat as for neuropathic pain.

NO ↓

GO TO PART 3

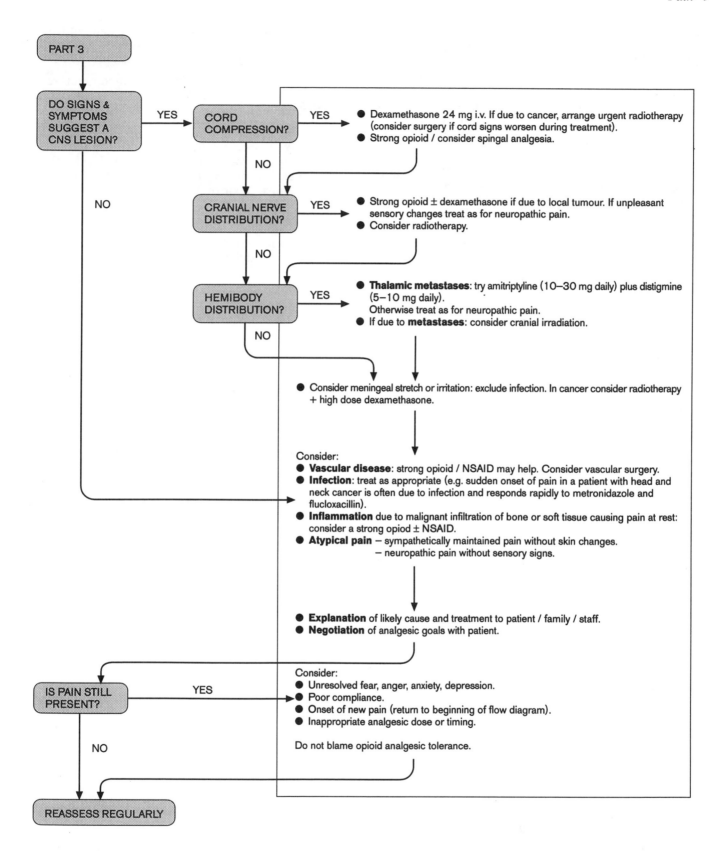

References

1. McNamara P, Minton M and Twycross RG. Use of midazolam in palliative care. *Palliative Medicine,* 1991; **5**: 244–49.

2. Swarm RA and Cousins MJ. Anaesthetic techniques for pain control. In: Doyle D, Hanks G and MacDonald N eds. *Oxford Textbook of Medicine*. Oxford: Oxford University Press 1993. pp. 204–221.

3. Sjöberg M, Nitescu, P, Appelgren L, Curelaru, I. Longterm intrathecal morphine and bupivacaine in patients with refractory cancer pain. *Anaesthesiology*, 1994; **80**: 284–297.

4. Ernst DS, MacDonald RN, Paterson AHG *et al* A double blind, cross-over trial of intravenous clodronate in metastatic bone pain. *J Pain Symp Manage,* 1992; **7**: 4–11.

5. Simons DG and Travell JG. Myofascial pain syndromes, In: Wall PD and Melzack R, eds, *Textbook of pain*, third edition. Edinburgh: Churchill Livingstone, 1994.

6. Thompson JW, Filshie J. TENS and acupuncture. In: Doyle D, Hanks G and MacDonald N., eds. *Oxford Textbook of Palliative Medicine*. Oxford: Oxford University Press, 1993. pp. 229–244.

7. Hanks GW, Portenoy RK, MacDonald N and O'Neill W. Difficult pain problems. In: Doyle D, Hanks G and MacDonald N., eds. *Oxford Textbook of Palliative Medicine*. Oxford: Oxford University Press, 1993. pp. 257–274.

8. Hampf G, Bowsher D and Nurmikko T. Distigmine and amitriptyline in the treatment of chronic pain. *Anaesth Prog* 1989; **36**: 58–62.

③ Constipation

Claud Regnard

Constipation is common in advanced disease and can cause many distressing symptoms. Prevention is the key, and the need to treat constipation is usually due to a failure of prevention. A rectal examination, using the correct technique, is an important part of the evaluation, and the action and appropriate use of laxatives should be understood. This flow diagram outlines the decisions and actions required to prevent and treat constipation.

Diagnosis

Constipation here is defined as the difficult or uncomfortable passage of faeces. In the absence of faeces, obstruction should be excluded. Accompanying symptoms are varied and include pain, anorexia, nausea, vomiting and diarrhoea. So called 'overflow diarrhoea' usually consists of small amounts of faecal fluid in the presence of an empty rectum. Accompanying signs are abdominal masses or distension and on occasions, faecal masses can be so hard and fixed that they are mistaken for tumours. A plain abdominal X-ray will clearly show the presence of faeces in the colon.

Rectal examination

This is an important part of assessment. It should be done slowly and gently with clear permission from the patient. The patient lies on their side, with knees drawn up. A lubricated gloved finger is placed *flat* with the finger pulp over the anus. Gentle pressure is applied on the posterior aspect of the anus. If this is done slowly, the anal sphincter will not contract, whilst the posterior pressure relaxes the pubo-rectalis muscle sling. The result is that the finger can be slipped slowly into the rectum with little or no discomfort. Withdrawal consists of the same actions in reverse.

Laxatives

Stimulant laxatives act mainly on the large bowel. Contact stimulant laxatives such as danthron, senna and bisacodyl act on the intestinal mucosa to increase the water content of faeces and enhance peristalsis. Danthron always colours the urine orange, brown or red, and can occasionally cause a perianal rash. Docusate is a weak contact stimulant, but with important surface wetting properties which is useful when softening stool is a priority, rather than stimulating its movement. Lactulose is an osmotic laxative which draws fluid into both the large and small bowel to soften stool and induce forward peristalsis, but it is expensive, and often causes bloating. It can also cause postural hypotension, even in well hydrated patients. Combinations of docusate and a contact stimulant often produce a comfortable stool. Co-danthrusate capsules (docusate and danthron) are often preferred to the sweet syrups of other combinations. A palatable alternative is senna and docusate in tablet form. The stimulant equivalents are shown in Table 1. Other types of laxatives need not be used. Laxatives should be taken on a regular basis with the dose adjusted every 3–5 days using stool consistency as the guide, not frequency.

Enemas

These are not often required. A high enema means slow delivery via a soft, suction- type catheter which has been gently inserted 10–15 cm into the rectum to prevent the contents being immediately expelled. Arachis oil given this way is more effective if it is left overnight and the foot of the bed is raised. A docusate enema is useful if hard stool is filling the rectum, since its surface wetting action will help to soften the stool.

Manual evacuations

Manual evacuations should be carried out under sedative cover such as diazepam or midazolam intravenously. Paraplegic patients do not usually require sedative cover and may need regular manual evacuations. This is easier if the faeces are kept firm and moved into the rectum by regular administration of a contact laxative acting mainly on the large bowel.

Managing constipation

A scheme for managing constipation should be based on a rational approach.[1] One approach is shown in this flow diagram.

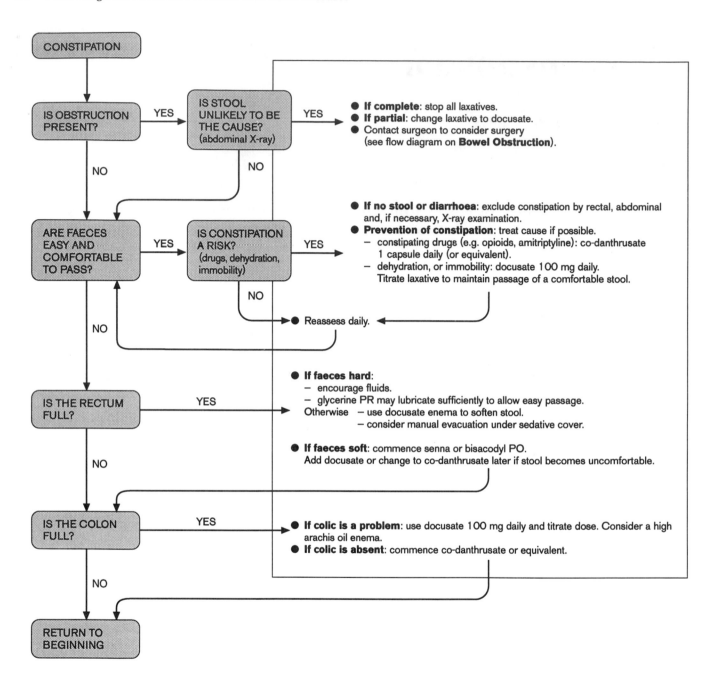

CONSTIPATION

IS OBSTRUCTION PRESENT? — YES → **IS STOOL UNLIKELY TO BE THE CAUSE?** (abdominal X-ray) — YES →
- **If complete**: stop all laxatives.
- **If partial**: change laxative to docusate.
- Contact surgeon to consider surgery (see flow diagram on **Bowel Obstruction**).

NO (from IS OBSTRUCTION PRESENT?)

NO (from IS STOOL UNLIKELY TO BE THE CAUSE?)

ARE FAECES EASY AND COMFORTABLE TO PASS? — YES → **IS CONSTIPATION A RISK?** (drugs, dehydration, immobility) — YES →
- **If no stool or diarrhoea**: exclude constipation by rectal, abdominal and, if necessary, X-ray examination.
- **Prevention of constipation**: treat cause if possible.
  - constipating drugs (e.g. opioids, amitriptyline): co-danthrusate 1 capsule daily (or equivalent).
  - dehydration, or immobility: docusate 100 mg daily. Titrate laxative to maintain passage of a comfortable stool.

NO (from IS CONSTIPATION A RISK?) → ● Reassess daily.

NO (from ARE FAECES EASY AND COMFORTABLE TO PASS?)

IS THE RECTUM FULL? — YES →
- **If faeces hard**:
  - encourage fluids.
  - glycerine PR may lubricate sufficiently to allow easy passage.
  Otherwise   – use docusate enema to soften stool.
              – consider manual evacuation under sedative cover.
- **If faeces soft**: commence senna or bisacodyl PO. Add docusate or change to co-danthrusate later if stool becomes uncomfortable.

NO (from IS THE RECTUM FULL?)

IS THE COLON FULL? — YES →
- **If colic is a problem**: use docusate 100 mg daily and titrate dose. Consider a high arachis oil enema.
- **If colic is absent**: commence co-danthrusate or equivalent.

NO (from IS THE COLON FULL?)

RETURN TO BEGINNING

Table 1 Contact stimulant laxatives

Approximate equivalents

Laxative	Preparation	Daily dose	Trade name
co-danthrusate	capsule	3	Normax
co-danthramer	sweet syrup	30 ml	Codalax
co-danthramer strong	sweet syrup	10 ml	Codalax Forte
senna and	tablet	2	Sennokot
docusate	tablet	200 mg	Dioctyl
senna and	sweet syrup	10 ml	Sennokot
lactulose	sweet syrup	10ml	Duphalac

Typical requirements for morphine-induced constipation

Oral morphine dose	Typical daily co-danthrusate dose
10 mg 4-hourly	2 capsules or equivalent
30 mg 4-hourly	4 capsules or equivalent
90 mg 4-hourly	6 capsules or equivalent

Adapted from: Constipation, In Regnard CFB, Tempest S. *A.*
Guide to Symptom Relief in Advanced Cancer, 3rd edition.
Manchester: Haigh and Hochland, 1992.

General care

If at all possible, patients should be given the dignity of being helped to the toilet since privacy will aid defaecation. Accurate, daily recordings of stool consistency, ease of defaecation and laxative administration are essential.

Reference

1. Sykes NP. Constipation and diarrhoea. In: Doyle D, Hanks G and MacDonald N., eds. *Oxford Textbook of Palliative Medicine*. Oxford: Oxford University Press, 1993. pp. 299–310.

4 Nausea and Vomiting

Claud Regnard
Mary Comiskey

Nausea and vomiting occur in many advanced diseases, and in far advanced cancer 42% of patients suffer nausea, 32% vomiting, with patients finding nausea almost as distressing as pain.[1] There are many causes, but successful treatment is possible in most patients when the clinician combines the history, symptoms, clinical examination and information about the patient's tumour, with existing knowledge about the mechanisms of nausea and vomiting. In this way antiemetics can be targeted at specific causes.

Causes of nausea and vomiting

Nausea and vomiting are the final common pathway of a variety of stimuli.[2] The vomiting centres in the medulla can be activated in the following ways.

Vagal stimulation can result from gastric distension, bowel distension, liver capsule·stretch, irritation of gastrointestinal mucosa (drugs, infection or radiotherapy), unpleasant genitourinary stimulation, or mediastinal disease.

Direct stimulation can arise from raised intracranial pressure, radiotherapy to the head and neck, or brain stem metastases.

Stimulation from the chemoreceptor trigger zone in the floor of the fourth ventricle can be caused by drugs (e.g. opioids, metronidazole, trimethoprim), bacterial toxins, and biochemical disturbances (hypercalcaemia, uraemia).

Stimulation from the inner or middle ear may be due to infection, movement, ototoxic drugs or local tumour.

Stimulation from higher central nervous system centres such as anxiety, fear, or revulsion.

Assessing the cause

History: it is useful to know the tumour histology (e.g. hypercalcaemia is commonest in myeloma, and in tumours of epithelial origin, especially breast and bronchus), tumour spread (e.g. intra-abdominal disease), previous treatment (e.g. past abdominal surgery), and current treatment (e.g. drugs). The pattern, speed of onset and association with drugs or with other symptoms may also provide clues.

Clinical features: Usually there are no clues as to the cause, with a non-specific pattern of nausea and vomiting. Accompanying symptoms may be helpful, such as symptoms of hypercalcaemia (drowsiness, confusion, constipation, thirst or polyuria; often only one symptom is present), or a history of abdominal distension in ascites. Gastric related causes are an important exception. Causes of altered gastric emptying tend to produce vomiting, preceded by mild or brief episodes of nausea, with sufficiently different features to differentiate each cause:

- Large volume vomiting suggests gastric stasis, and is often accompanied by symptoms such as oesophageal reflux, epigastric fullness, early satiation or hiccups. Gastric stasis may be caused by reduced motility due to drugs (although there is still enough gastric tone to vomit), or due to partial outflow obstruction caused by local tumour (e.g. pancreatic carcinoma, hepatomegaly, ascites, abdominal tumour).
- Repeated, forceful vomiting with rapid dehydration suggests total gastric outflow obstruction, an uncommon cause of vomiting.
- Symptoms of gastric stasis, but with low volume vomiting, suggests a 'squashed stomach syndrome'. In this syndrome there is no outflow obstruction, but the stomach is compressed externally by tumour, ascites or hepatomegaly, or the stomach lumen is reduced by carcinoma. Occasionally gastric tone is virtually absent, resulting in a stomach grossly distended by fluid, air or both. In this 'floppy stomach syndrome' only small volume vomiting occurs, with variable amounts of nausea. The cause may be gastric atony due to autonomic failure,[3] and seems to occur more commonly in some patients in their last days of life.
- Regurgitation due to a swallowing disorder is suggested by a history of small 'vomits' of food or fluid ingested within the last hour.

Examination and investigation: Abdominal examination is essential and may reveal constipation, hepatomegaly, ascites, some tumour masses, gastric or bowel distension. Auscultation can provide a rough guide to bowel motility. Fundoscopy (to exclude papilloedema) and oropharyngeal

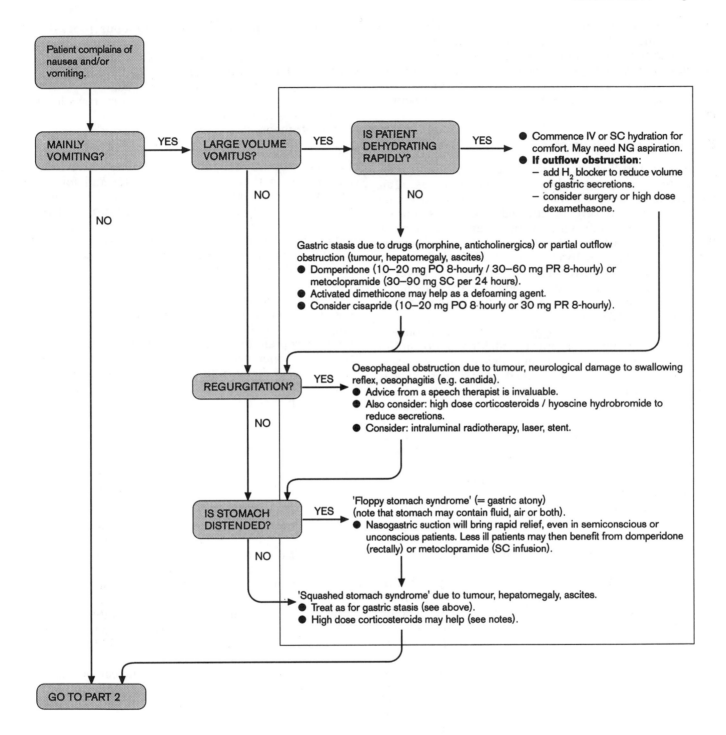

examination may also help. For any unexplained nausea and vomiting, and if treatment is appropriate, it is necessary to check the serum urea, calcium (corrected for albumin) and electrolyte levels. Finally, in regurgitation, a simple litmus test of the vomitus will distinguish the lack of acid content from a blockage above the oesophageal sphincter.

Choosing an antiemetic

From animal studies there is evidence of a concentration of histamine receptors in the vomiting centres, making an antihistamine drug a logical choice in causes affecting these centres directly or through the vagus nerve.[4] Cyclizine is an antihistamine with antiemetic properties that is often effective in direct, or vagally mediated causes. Although the vagal pathway is mediated through acetylcholine, the potent anticholinergic hyoscine hydrobromide (scopolamine) tends to have a high adverse effect profile, but is still useful as second line treatment to cyclizine.

At the chemoreceptor trigger zone there is a concentration of dopamine receptors, making a dopamine antagonist a logical choice for chemical causes of nausea and vomiting.[4] Haloperidol is the drug of choice, since it is potent and has a long action (a half life of approximately 16 hours) so that a dose of 1.5–3 mg once at night is sufficient for most patients, resulting in few adverse effects. Metoclopramide has little central antiemetic action; prochlorperazine has an unpredictable oral absorption rate; chlorpromazine and methotrimeprazine are less potent dopamine antagonists, but are too sedating for some patients.

Peripheral dopamine receptors are present in the stomach and upper small bowel. Domperidone and metoclopramide will normalise upper gastrointestinal motility, making them useful in gastric-related syndromes. Domperidone is approximately 30% more expensive but has a lower adverse effect profile. It is not available in injectable form, although it is available in suppository form. Methotrimeprazine and chlorpromazine should be avoided in these patients, since their anticholinergic action may precipitate or worsen gastric stasis. Cisapride is a useful second line agent in gastric stasis because of its more extensive stimulation of gastrointestinal motility, but is approximately five times the cost of metoclopramide.

Some patients have more than one cause of nausea and vomiting (e.g. gastric stasis and hypercalcaemia), requiring two antiemetics (e.g. domperidone plus haloperidol). With the above regimen only one third of patients will require more than one antiemetic,[5] and the scheme has been shown to be effective in 93% of patients with advanced disease.[6]

Methotrimeprazine has a role in the small number of patients who fail on the above regimen. Low doses are often sufficient (25–75 mg daily), and avoid the sedation and hypotension seen with higher doses.

The five antiemetics recommended above are most usefully given by the following routes:

- cyclizine – oral, rectal, subcutaneous (occasional irritation).
- haloperidol – oral, subcutaneous.
- domperidone – oral, rectal.
- metoclopramide – oral, subcutaneous.
- hyoscine hydrobromide – oral, sublingual, transdermal.
- cisapride – oral, rectal.
- methotrimepruzine – oral, subcutaneous.

Ondansetron and granisetron are the first of a new class of antiemetic, the $5HT_3$ antagonists. They have proven value in chemotherapy-induced emesis and following bowel irradiation, but to date have been disappointing when used in causes of nausea and vomiting that have failed on the above scheme. It is not known whether they would be more effective in combination with the antiemetics in this scheme, but their high cost and low efficacy used alone in advanced disease make their place in palliative care unclear.

For subcutaneous infusions, compatibility should not be assumed on visual inspection alone. Diamorphine is compatible with haloperidol, hyoscine hydrobromide, and metoclopramide.[7] Cyclizine can precipitate or crystalise if the concentration of either drug is above 20 mg/ml,[8] but higher diamorphine concentrations can be used if the cyclizine concentration is no higher than 10 mg/ml.[7] A sensible rule is to mix no more than two drugs in one syringe.

Associated management

Nasogastric suction: It is unusual to use nasogastric suction in palliative care, but there are several exceptions:

- Total gastric outflow obstruction, where improved comfort can be achieved using nasogastric suction to reduce gastric distension. The use of H_2 blockers will reduce the volume of gastric secretions.
- Floppy stomach syndrome, where nasogastric suction will stop restlessness due to distension, and prevents the release of a large volume of gastric contents through the mouth at the time of death, which can cause considerable distress to those present. In semiconscious or unconscious patients a tube is often easily passed with little or no discomfort and can be removed once all fluid and air have been aspirated.
- Faeculant or faecal vomiting (see the flow diagram on *Bowel Obstruction*).

Parenteral hydration is accepted practice in two palliative care situations, as part of the treatment of hypercalcaemia, and in severe gastric outflow obstruction. Common to both these situations is rapid dehydration over 24–36 hours, causing thirst, hypotension and lethargy. Rapid dehydration can also occur because of repeated vomiting from other causes, making this a third indication for parenteral hydration, with comfort as the aim. A fourth indication may be patients with a hyperactive confusional state (see also the flow diagram on *Reduced Hydration and Feeding*).

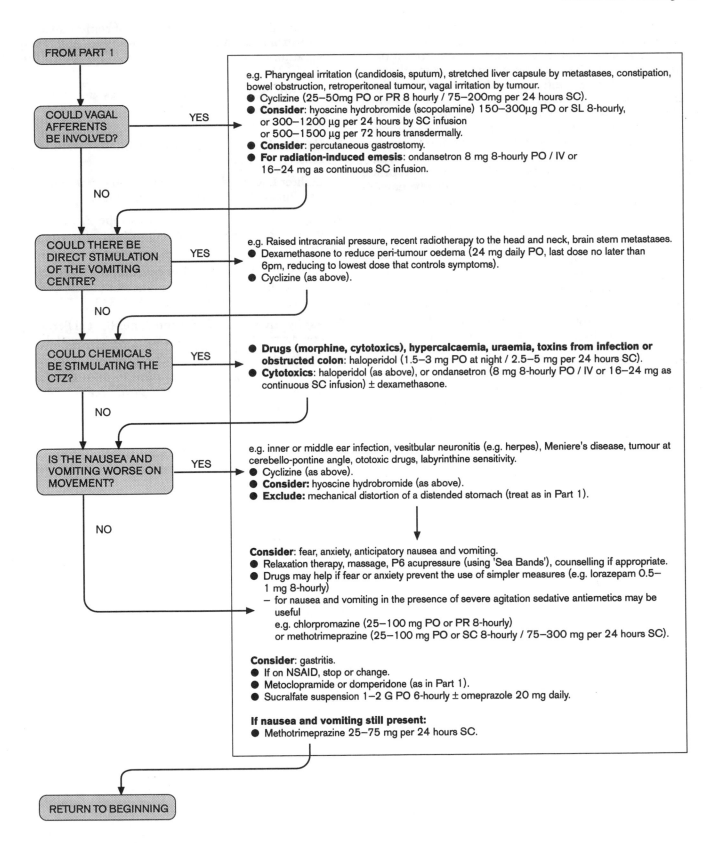

FROM PART 1

COULD VAGAL AFFERENTS BE INVOLVED? — YES →

e.g. Pharyngeal irritation (candidosis, sputum), stretched liver capsule by metastases, constipation, bowel obstruction, retroperitoneal tumour, vagal irritation by tumour.
● Cyclizine (25–50mg PO or PR 8 hourly / 75–200mg per 24 hours SC).
● **Consider**: hyoscine hydrobromide (scopolamine) 150–300μg PO or SL 8-hourly, or 300–1200 μg per 24 hours by SC infusion or 500–1500 μg per 72 hours transdermally.
● **Consider**: percutaneous gastrostomy.
● **For radiation-induced emesis**: ondansetron 8 mg 8-hourly PO / IV or 16–24 mg as continuous SC infusion.

NO ↓

COULD THERE BE DIRECT STIMULATION OF THE VOMITING CENTRE? — YES →

e.g. Raised intracranial pressure, recent radiotherapy to the head and neck, brain stem metastases.
● Dexamethasone to reduce peri-tumour oedema (24 mg daily PO, last dose no later than 6pm, reducing to lowest dose that controls symptoms).
● Cyclizine (as above).

NO ↓

COULD CHEMICALS BE STIMULATING THE CTZ? — YES →

● **Drugs (morphine, cytotoxics), hypercalcaemia, uraemia, toxins from infection or obstructed colon**: haloperidol (1.5–3 mg PO at night / 2.5–5 mg per 24 hours SC).
● **Cytotoxics**: haloperidol (as above), or ondansetron (8 mg 8-hourly PO / IV or 16–24 mg as continuous SC infusion) ± dexamethasone.

NO ↓

IS THE NAUSEA AND VOMITING WORSE ON MOVEMENT? — YES →

e.g. inner or middle ear infection, vesitbular neuronitis (e.g. herpes), Meniere's disease, tumour at cerebello-pontine angle, ototoxic drugs, labyrinthine sensitivity.
● Cyclizine (as above).
● **Consider:** hyoscine hydrobromide (as above).
● **Exclude:** mechanical distortion of a distended stomach (treat as in Part 1).

↓

Consider: fear, anxiety, anticipatory nausea and vomiting.
● Relaxation therapy, massage, P6 acupressure (using 'Sea Bands'), counselling if appropriate.
● Drugs may help if fear or anxiety prevent the use of simpler measures (e.g. lorazepam 0.5–1 mg 8-hourly)
  – for nausea and vomiting in the presence of severe agitation sedative antiemetics may be useful
    e.g. chlorpromazine (25–100 mg PO or PR 8-hourly)
    or methotrimeprazine (25–100 mg PO or SC 8-hourly / 75–300 mg per 24 hours SC).

Consider: gastritis.
● If on NSAID, stop or change.
● Metoclopramide or domperidone (as in Part 1).
● Sucralfate suspension 1–2 G PO 6-hourly ± omeprazole 20 mg daily.

If nausea and vomiting still present:
● Methotrimeprazine 25–75 mg per 24 hours SC.

NO ↓

RETURN TO BEGINNING

Other approaches: Patients with gastric stasis can benefit from activated dimethicone (in Asilone, Windcheaters) which acts as a defoaming agent and helps gastric air to be brought up. High dose corticosteroids (dexamethasone 24 mg daily PO or SC infusion, reducing to 4–8mg daily over 10 days) by reducing peritumour oedema may open the lumen in gastric outflow obstruction or relieve compression in squashed stomach syndrome due to tumour or hepatomegaly. Nausea and vomiting due to tumour pressure may be amenable to radiotherapy, chemotherapy or laser, and these should be considered in appropriate patients. Percutaneous gastrostomy can also be considered.[9] Effective mouth care is essential, especially if the patient is vomiting (see flow diagram on *Mouth Care*). Anxiety and fear should be approached as usual, but simple measures such as relaxation, massage, or pressure over the P6 acupuncture point[10] using 'Sea Bands' can be helpful. Severe agitation may require a sedative antiemetic such as chlorpromazine or methotrimeprazine. Finally gastric irritation (stress ulceration, drug irritation) can be helped by sucralfate suspension, with the optional addition of omeprazole or an H_2 blocker.

References

1. Dunlop GM. A study of the relative frequency and importance of gastrointestinal symptoms and weakness in patients with far-advanced cancer. *Palliative Medicine*, 1989; **4**: 37–43.

2. Allan SG. Nausea and vomiting. In: Doyle D, Hanks G and MacDonald N eds. *Oxford Textbook of Palliative Medicine*. Oxford: Oxford University Press 1993. pp. 282 – 290.

3. Bruera E, Catz Z, Hooper et al Chronic nausea and anorexia in advanced cancer patients: a possible role for autonomic dysfunction. *J Pain Symp Manag* 1987; **2**: 19–21.

4. Peroutka SJ, Snyder SH. Antiemetics: neurotransmitter receptor binding predicts therapeutic actions. *Lancet*, 1982; **i**: 658–659.

5. Hanks GW. Antiemetics for terminal cancer patients. *Lancet*, 1982; **i**: 1410.

6. Lichter I. Results of antiemetic management in terminal illness. *J Pall Care* 1993; **9**: 19–21.

7. Regnard C, Pashley S and Westrope F. Antiemetic/diamorphine mixture compatibility in infusion pumps. *Br J Pharm Pract*, 1986; **8**: 218–220.

8. Allwood MC. The stability of diamorphine alone and in combination with antiemetics in plastic syringes. *Palliative Medicine*, 1991; **5**: 330–333.

9. Ashby MA, Game PA, Britten-Jones R, et al Percutaneous gastrostomy as a venting procedure. *Palliative Medicine*, 1991; **5**: 147–150.

10. Dundee JW, McMillan C. Positive evidence for P6 acupuncture antiemesis. *Postgrad Med J*, 1991; **67**: 417–422.

5 Dysphagia

Claud Regnard

Dysphagia is very common in motor neurone disease and can occur in up to 83% of head and neck cancer patients,[1] but can also occur in any cancers involving the mediastinum, such as in the oesophagus and bronchus, and in infections involving the mucosa. Dysphagia is here defined as difficulty in transferring solids, pastes or liquids from the oral cavity to the stomach in patients with advanced disease. This flow diagram outlines the clinical steps required to manage dysphagia when hydration and feeding are appropriate, and explains the importance of including a swallowing therapist in these decisions.

Causes

There are many problems that can alter the complex anatomy and physiology of swallowing. It is therefore important to understand the normal process, and complete a careful assessment of the cause before treatment can start. Oral disorders may affect the preparatory phase of swallowing and delay or prevent initiation of the oral swallowing phase. Most disorders of the pharynx and difficulty with laryngeal closure will affect the pharyngeal phase of swallowing. The oesophageal phase will be affected by oesophageal problems. Causes may be direct (such as cancer causing luminal, intramural or extramural obstruction), or indirect (such as neurological deficits in motor neurone disease or cranial nerve damage due to cancer). Treatment may affect swallowing after surgery (altered anatomy, fibrosis, fistula, neurological damage), radiotherapy (dryness, inflammation, fibrosis, necrosis) or chemotherapy (mucosal ulceration, zoster). Debility can allow infections (candida, herpes, zoster), or result in drowsiness and extreme weakness.

Evaluation

The advice of a swallowing therapist (often a speech therapist with a specialist interest) can be invaluable at this stage. Although localisation by the patient corresponds to the anatomical site of the problem in 99% of patients, difficulties with certain food consistencies is much less reliable.[2] Symptoms suggesting aspiration are important: choking, coughing, copious secretions, frequent chest infections. The site of the pain may help localise the pathology: for example pain referred to the ear suggests a tumour of the pyriform fossae, base of the tongue, vallecula or mediastinal tumour.

Examination at the bedside will identify problems with oral preparatory and oral swallowing phases. A test swallow will allow an estimate to be made of the oral-pharyngeal transit time (the time from the first movement of the tongue base, to the last movement of the larynx) – times of more than one second are abnormal. Speaking at the end of swallowing may detect a 'gargle' quality to the voice, suggesting (in the absence of coughing or choking) silent aspiration. Accurate investigation of the pharyngeal and oesophageal phases can only be done radiologically. This is particularly important if aspiration is suspected, since the extent of aspiration dictates management. In addition, bedside examination will uncover aspiration in only 60% of cases.[2]

Management

It is necessary for the team to assess the need for hydration and feeding and, if possible, to discuss this with the patient. In the last days of a patient's life hydration and feeding are often inappropriate, but it can be difficult for some staff and relatives to separate eating for survival from drinking for pleasure or comfort. Both need support in understanding this (see also the flow diagram on *Reduced Hydration and Feeding*). If hydration and feeding are appropriate, however, then proceed as in the flow diagram.

Complete obstruction will require parenteral hydration with or without feeding, with assessment for removing the obstruction or opening the lumen. Oral problems should be treated appropriately. Some drugs can exacerbate swallowing problems and should be stopped or replaced. Pain related to swallowing should be treated appropriately. Patients should also be considered for radiotherapy, surgery, laser, or chemotherapy if these are appropriate. Single dose, intraluminal irradiation of oesophageal carcinoma can relieve dysphagia in up to 70% of patients for as long as 50 weeks.[3] Endoscopic entubation of oesophageal tumours is an alternative and simple procedure.[4] Peritumour oedema due to soft tissue infection should be treated with appropriate antibiotics. In the absence of such infection, high dose corticosteroids may offer the possibility of reopening the lumen.

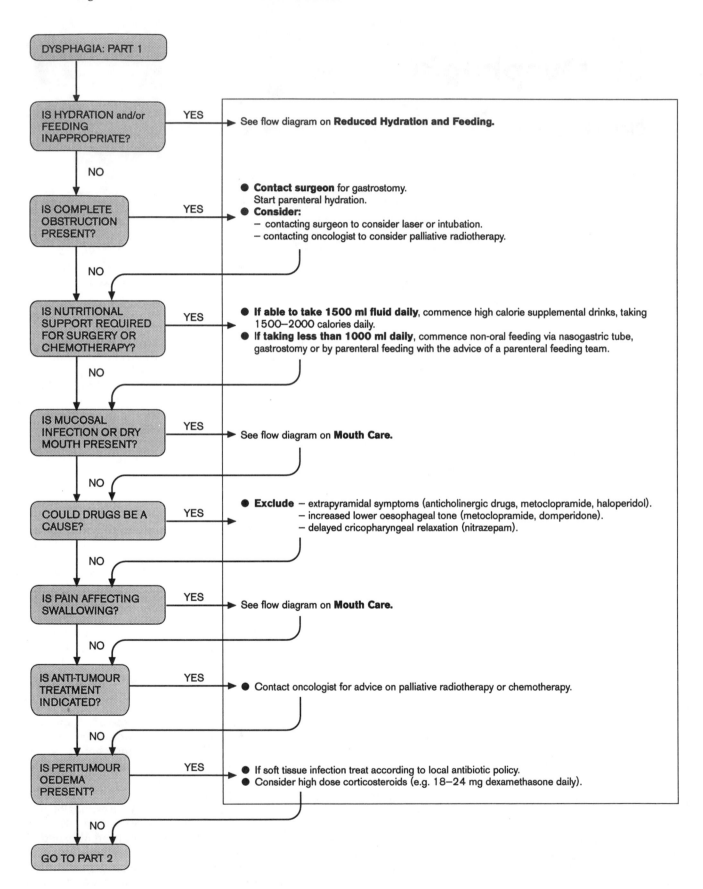

DYSPHAGIA: PART 1

IS HYDRATION and/or FEEDING INAPPROPRIATE?
YES → See flow diagram on **Reduced Hydration and Feeding.**

NO

IS COMPLETE OBSTRUCTION PRESENT?
YES →
- **Contact surgeon** for gastrostomy. Start parenteral hydration.
- **Consider:**
  - contacting surgeon to consider laser or intubation.
  - contacting oncologist to consider palliative radiotherapy.

NO

IS NUTRITIONAL SUPPORT REQUIRED FOR SURGERY OR CHEMOTHERAPY?
YES →
- **If able to take 1500 ml fluid daily**, commence high calorie supplemental drinks, taking 1500–2000 calories daily.
- **If taking less than 1000 ml daily**, commence non-oral feeding via nasogastric tube, gastrostomy or by parenteral feeding with the advice of a parenteral feeding team.

NO

IS MUCOSAL INFECTION OR DRY MOUTH PRESENT?
YES → See flow diagram on **Mouth Care.**

NO

COULD DRUGS BE A CAUSE?
YES →
- **Exclude** – extrapyramidal symptoms (anticholinergic drugs, metoclopramide, haloperidol).
  - increased lower oesophageal tone (metoclopramide, domperidone).
  - delayed cricopharyngeal relaxation (nitrazepam).

NO

IS PAIN AFFECTING SWALLOWING?
YES → See flow diagram on **Mouth Care.**

NO

IS ANTI-TUMOUR TREATMENT INDICATED?
YES →
- Contact oncologist for advice on palliative radiotherapy or chemotherapy.

NO

IS PERITUMOUR OEDEMA PRESENT?
YES →
- If soft tissue infection treat according to local antibiotic policy.
- Consider high dose corticosteroids (e.g. 18–24 mg dexamethasone daily).

NO

GO TO PART 2

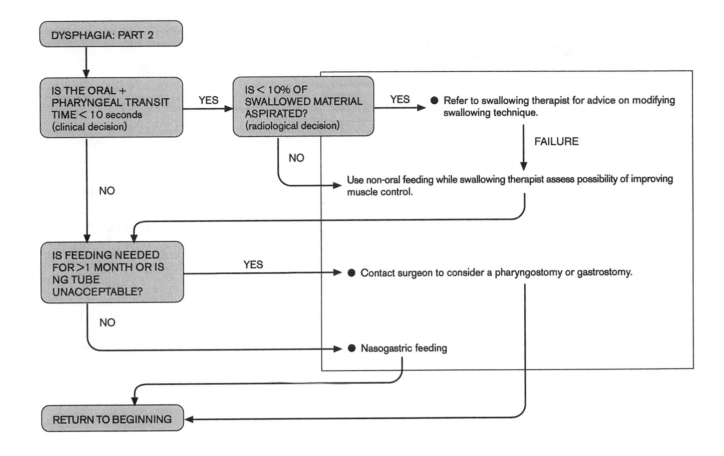

Patients tend to reject certain food consistencies if they find it takes too long to swallow. This is likely to occur when the oral-pharyngeal transit time is more than 10 seconds. It will then be necessary to consider non-oral feeding with the advice of a swallowing therapist. Short term feeding is acceptable through fine bore nasogastric tubes which are well tolerated. For some patients, however, such tubes are cosmetically unacceptable and if feeding is likely to be required for more than one month an alternative route is required. A pharyngostomy provides safe, simple access and can be fashioned under a local anaesthetic if necessary.[5] Alternatively a percutaneous gastrostomy can be used.[6] Great care needs to be taken of the skin surrounding the gastrostomy site, since any irritation can become a painful and difficult problem. Karya gum products will provide adequate protection.

If the oral-pharyngeal transit time is less than 10 seconds and less than 10% of swallowed material is aspirated, then it may be possible to modify the swallowing technique. There are many such techniques; for example patients with reduced laryngeal closure are helped by the supraglottic swallow:

- hold the breath
- place the food in the mouth
- tilt the head back and swallow
- cough.

Patients who are not helped by swallowing techniques, or who aspirate more than 10% of swallowed material will require non-oral feeding while they are assessed for possibilities of improving muscle control.

References

1. Robertson MS and Hornibrook J. The presenting symptoms of head and neck cancer. *NZ Med J,* 1982; **95**: 337–41.

2. Logemann JA. In: *Evaluation and treatment of Swallowing Disorders*. San Diego: College Hill Press, 1983.

3. Rowland CG and Pagliero KM. Intracavity irradiation of carcinoma of oesophagus and cardia. *Lancet*, 1985; *ii*: 981–3.

4. Pfleiderer AG, Goodall P and Holmes GKT. The consequences and effectiveness of intubation in the palliation of dysphagia due to benign and malignant strictures affecting the oesophagus. *Br J Surg*, 1982; **69**: 356-8.

5. Meehan SE, Wood RAB and Cuschieri A. Percutaneous cervical pharyngostomy: a comfortable and convenient alternative to protracted nasogastric intubation. *Am J Surg,* 1984; **148**: 325- 30.

6. Ashby MA, Game PA, Britten-Jones *et al*. Percutaneous gastrostomy as a venting procedure. *Palliative Medicine* 1991; **5**: 147-50.

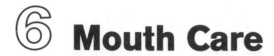

⑥ Mouth Care

Claud Regnard
Sarah Fitton

Oral problems are common in advanced disease and regular mouth care is essential. Ulceration, oral debris, dryness and pain each have to be managed in turn. This flow diagram outlines the decisions and actions required to achieve a clean, moist, pain free mouth.

Prevention

Regular mouth care is essential to prevent oral problems. Risk factors include debility, reduced oral intake (due to anorexia, nausea, vomiting, dysphagia, local tumour, weakness, odour etc.) anticholinergic drugs, local irradiation, malignant ulceration, chemotherapy and dehydration. Patients at risk will require frequent (up to hourly) care with an antibacterial and antifungal mouth wash. Good dental care is essential and the support of an understanding dentist is invaluable.[1]

Infection

Zoster or herpes simplex infections will cause ulceration and pain. If severe, they will require systemic acyclovir. Multiple apthous ulcers can be helped with 250 mg tetracycline (the contents of one capsule stirred in water) as a 2 minute mouth wash every 8 hours. Persistent apthous ulceration in AIDS has been reported to respond to thalidomide.[2] Infection associated with malignant ulceration may require systemic antibiotics if soft tissue infection is suspected. Foul odours are usually associated with anaerobic infections, which may respond to metronidazole. This can be applied topically if not tolerated systemically – there is no indication for giving other antibiotics topically.

Oral candida most commonly presents with white adherent patches, angular chelitis (inflammation at the angles of the mouth), redness or soreness. Many cases may be due to an overgrowth in immunocompromised patients, since cross infection does not occur easily. Topical antifungals (e.g. nystatin) are effective, but they do not clear candida harbouring in dentures. Non-metal dentures are best cleaned in weak chlorine releasing solutions (e.g. 1% sodium hypochlorite, Eusol, Dakin's) and metal dentures in nystatin. Ketoconazole is a systemic antifungal and is effective at a dose of 200 mg daily for 5 days.[3] Nystatin and miconazole are much less convenient to the patient and more expensive. The incidence of potentially serious hepatic injury with ketoconazole is low (1 in 15 000 exposed individuals)[4] and should not preclude its use for short courses. An alternative, more expensive, but very convenient option is fluconoazole as a single dose of 150mg.[3] Prophylactic antifungals do not reduce the proportion of positive mouth swabs,[5] but in debilitated patients overt infection persists and treatment for longer than one week may be necessary. For prophylaxis, fluconazole is usually used at a dose of 50 mg on alternate days. Fluconazole is also the antifungal of choice in AIDS, where the occurrence of reduced gastric acidity will reduce the absorption of ketoconazole.

Dirty mouth

Once infection has been treated or excluded, the removal of adherent debris may be helped by effervescent solutions such as cider and soda water. Hydrogen peroxide tends to foam too rapidly for some patients and has the disadvantage that it damages granulating tissue. An alternative is chewing unsweetened pineapple chunks which contain a proteolytic enzyme, annanase which helps to remove adherent coatings.[6] Annanase remains fully active in tinned pineapple. Sodium bicarbonate 2% can be used but has an unpleasant taste and may damage the mucosa.[7] Cleaning a coated tongue with a cleansing solution is helped by the gentle use of a soft or baby toothbrush.[8] Removal of oral debris can be helped by irrigation with a warm solution, which is soothing and non-traumatic. Higginson's syringes can be used for this purpose. Further debridement can be done with foam-covered sticks soaked in a cleansing solution or the gentle use of a gloved hand and soaked swab.

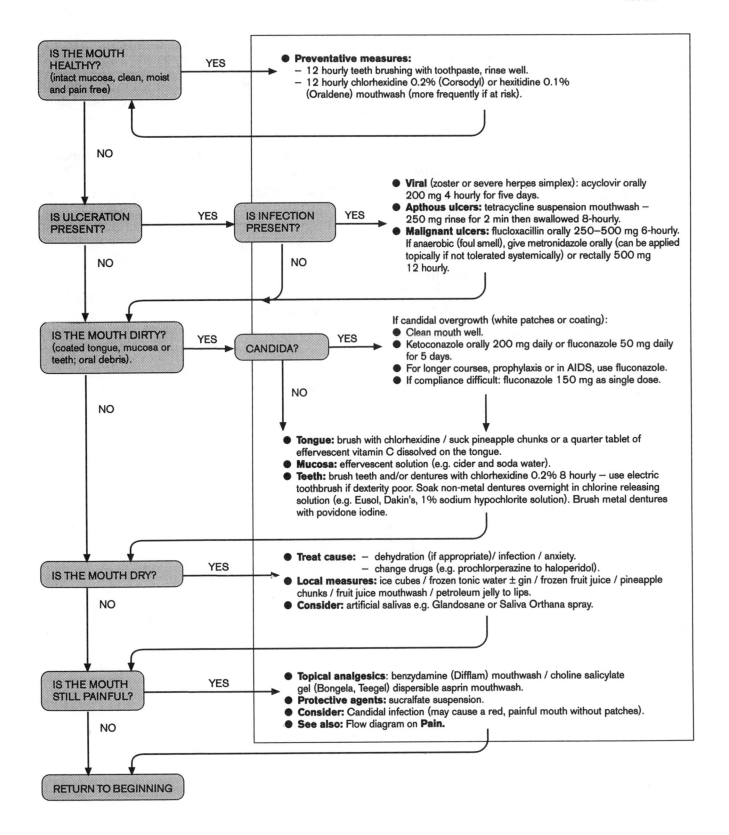

IS THE MOUTH HEALTHY?
(intact mucosa, clean, moist and pain free)

YES →
- **Preventative measures:**
  - 12 hourly teeth brushing with toothpaste, rinse well.
  - 12 hourly chlorhexidine 0.2% (Corsodyl) or hexitidine 0.1% (Oraldene) mouthwash (more frequently if at risk).

NO ↓

IS ULCERATION PRESENT?

YES → **IS INFECTION PRESENT?**

YES →
- **Viral** (zoster or severe herpes simplex): acyclovir orally 200 mg 4 hourly for five days.
- **Apthous ulcers:** tetracycline suspension mouthwash – 250 mg rinse for 2 min then swallowed 8-hourly.
- **Malignant ulcers:** flucloxacillin orally 250–500 mg 6-hourly. If anaerobic (foul smell), give metronidazole orally (can be applied topically if not tolerated systemically) or rectally 500 mg 12 hourly.

NO (under IS ULCERATION PRESENT?) ↓

NO (under IS INFECTION PRESENT?) ↓

IS THE MOUTH DIRTY?
(coated tongue, mucosa or teeth; oral debris).

YES → **CANDIDA?**

YES →
If candidal overgrowth (white patches or coating):
- Clean mouth well.
- Ketoconazole orally 200 mg daily or fluconazole 50 mg daily for 5 days.
- For longer courses, prophylaxis or in AIDS, use fluconazole.
- If compliance difficult: fluconazole 150 mg as single dose.

NO (under CANDIDA?) ↓

- **Tongue:** brush with chlorhexidine / suck pineapple chunks or a quarter tablet of effervescent vitamin C dissolved on the tongue.
- **Mucosa:** effervescent solution (e.g. cider and soda water).
- **Teeth:** brush teeth and/or dentures with chlorhexidine 0.2% 8 hourly – use electric toothbrush if dexterity poor. Soak non-metal dentures overnight in chlorine releasing solution (e.g. Eusol, Dakin's, 1% sodium hypochlorite solution). Brush metal dentures with povidone iodine.

NO (under IS THE MOUTH DIRTY?) ↓

IS THE MOUTH DRY?

YES →
- **Treat cause:** – dehydration (if appropriate)/ infection / anxiety.
  – change drugs (e.g. prochlorperazine to haloperidol).
- **Local measures:** ice cubes / frozen tonic water ± gin / frozen fruit juice / pineapple chunks / fruit juice mouthwash / petroleum jelly to lips.
- **Consider:** artificial salivas e.g. Glandosane or Saliva Orthana spray.

NO ↓

IS THE MOUTH STILL PAINFUL?

YES →
- **Topical analgesics:** benzydamine (Difflam) mouthwash / choline salicylate gel (Bongela, Teegel) dispersible asprin mouthwash.
- **Protective agents:** sucralfate suspension.
- **Consider:** Candidal infection (may cause a red, painful mouth without patches).
- **See also:** Flow diagram on **Pain.**

NO ↓

RETURN TO BEGINNING

Dry mouth

It may be appropriate to treat the cause. Hypercalcaemic dehydration is usually easily treated. Drugs that cause a dry mouth (e.g. anticholinergics) should be reviewed since they may be changed to drugs less likely to cause this problem (e.g. prochlorperazine to haloperidol; amitriptyline to lofepramine). When it is inappropriate or impossible to treat the cause (e.g. terminal dehydration or salivary gland destruction) local measures can be tried. Petroleum jelly to the lips, fruit juice mouthwashes, sucking frozen tonic water, frozen fruit juice, frozen whisky and lemonade, and chewing pineapple chunks may all be helpful. Mouth care every 1–2 hours may be necessary. Artificial salivas containing methylcellulose have an oily taste, although some sprays (e.g. Glandosane) are well received by patients. A very effective alternative is a mucin spray (Saliva Orthana), although its porcine source will prevent its use in some patients on religious grounds. Artificial salivas may have to be used several times each hour to be effective. Glycerin has a dehydrating effects on the mucosa,[9] and should be avoided. Lemon juice stimulates salivary flow but can soon cause exhaustion of the salivary glands with frequent use.[8]

Painful mouth

If pain is not due to infection, then the source may be mucosa, bone, soft tissue or nerve. Pain from the mucosa may be helped by topical analgesics such as choline salicylate gel (Bonjela, Teejel). Benzydamine (Difflam) is a topical nonsteroidal antiinflammatory drug used a mouthwash every 1–2 hours, but which produces some local numbness. Pain due to widespread ulceration caused by chemotherapy or other causes is eased with sucralfate suspension as a mouthwash.[10] Local anaesthetics (lignocaine, benzocaine) will result in unpleasant numbness, which may prevent safe eating and drinking, and their place is limited to use before painful procedures. Other causes of pain should be managed as outlined in the flow diagram on *Pain*.

General care

When patients are unable to manage their own mouth care, it must be done regularly by the nurse, relative or partner. Using a gloved finger and a moistened gauze to clean the mouth is the simplest and most effective method.

References

1. Walls AWG and Murray ID. Dental care of patients in a hospice. *Palliative Medicine* 1993; **7**: 313–321.

2. Youle M, Clarbour J, Farthing C *et al*. Treatment of resistant apthous ulceration with thalidomide in patients positive for HIV antibody. *BMJ* 1989; **298**: 432.

3. Regnard C. Single dose fluconazole versus five day ketoconazole in oral candidiasis. *Palliative Medicine* 1994; **8**: 72–73.

4. Hay RJ. Ketoconazole: a reappraisal. *Br Med J* 1985; **290**: 260–261.

5. Finlay IG. Oral symptoms and candida in the terminally ill. *Br Med J*, 1986; **292**: 592-593.

6. Twycross RG and Lack SA. The mouth, In: *Control of Alimentary Symptoms in Far Advanced Cancer*, 1986. Edinburgh: Churchill Livingstone.

7. Eds Pritchard P, Walker VA. Mouth Care, In: *Manual of Clinical Nursing Policies and Procedures: The Royal Marsden Hospital*, 1984. London: Harper & Row.

8. Sammon P, Page C and Shepherd G. Oral Hygiene. *Nursing Times*, 1987; **83**: 25-27.

9. Van Drimmelen J and Rollins HF. Evaluation of a commonly used oral hygiene agent. *Nursing Research*, 1969; **18**: 327-332.

10. Solomon MA. Oral sucralfate suspension for mucositis. *N Eng J Med* 1986; **4**: 29-32.

7 Reduced Hydration or Feeding

Claud Regnard
Kathryn Mannix

Reduced hydration and feeding are here defined as a reduction in the intake and quality of drink or food sufficient to produce weight loss, nutritional deficiency, or both. This flow diagram outlines the management of reversible and irreversible causes of reduced intake.

When hydration and feeding are no longer appropriate

In patients with a short prognosis (day to day deterioration) hydration and feeding may become unnecessary. At the end of life some dehydration is not distressing and has the advantages of reduced urinary output, absence of bronchial secretions and reduction or cessation of vomiting. Dehydration is normal at the end of life. It can be difficult, however, for some staff and families to accept this situation, and they may need support and counselling to understand that hydration and feeding now only need be for pleasure or local oral comfort.

If the prognosis is longer (week to week, or month to month deterioration), then proceed as follows.

When hydration and feeding are appropriate

Exclude psychological or psychiatric cause: psychological withdrawal or anxiety can result in reduced intake. For the management see the flow diagrams *Managing the Withdrawn Patient*, and *Managing the Anxious Patient*.

Leaving the intake unchanged: Once psychological causes are excluded, the patient may be content with the present low intake, or ask for it to remain at a low level. For example, they may not realise the need for adequate nutrition when this would be helpful, or they may mistakenly believe that adequate nutrition will prolong their lives. In this situation mouth and skin care are important (see the flow diagrams on *Mouth Care* and *Pressure Sores*).

Swallowing difficulties may be due to oral problems which should be treated appropriately (see flow diagram on *Mouth Care*), or to problems with the other phases of swallowing. In some patients it may be appropriate to consider a feeding pharyngostomy or endoscopically placed gastrostomy tube. Indications for choosing a non-oral feeding route are: a prolonged oral-pharyngeal transit time; failure to modify swallowing technique; during exercises to improve swallowing control or for nutritional support prior to surgery or chemotherapy.[1] Contraindications include rapid deterioration, and dysphagia due to exhaustion, debility or weakness caused by the advanced disease. When these decisions are being made the advice of a speech therapist with an interest in swallowing disorders is invaluable. For more details see the flow diagram on *Dysphagia*.

If the patient is weak or disabled: Some patients (e.g. those suffering from advanced motor neurone disease, or exhaustion) may be too disabled to feed themselves and they need regular help. If present at rest, dyspnoea will reduce intake and the associated anxiety will reduce appetite. Treatment of dyspnoea will depend on the cause (see the flow diagram on *Dyspnoea*).

Gastrointestinal problems: Intake is invariably reduced in bowel obstruction, but it is often possible for patients to continue with some oral hydration and feeding (see flow diagram on *Bowel Obstruction*). Constipation will reduce the appetite, as will nausea and vomiting. Constipation should be prevented in at risk patients (e.g. opioids, reduced mobility) with regular, prophylactic laxatives (see the flow diagram on *Constipation*). Nausea and vomiting will need treatment with appropriately selected drugs (see the flow diagram on *Nausea and Vomiting*).

Infection from most sources will reduce the appetite and should be treated when appropriate. Odour is distressing and will reduce the appetite of the patient involved and of surrounding patients. Odours should be cleared with adequate ventilation as soon as they occur. The source of odours should be treated or masked (see the flow diagram on *Malignant Ulcers*).

Drugs can reduce the appetite by causing nausea, mucosal irritation, delayed gastric emptying or central suppression. Often the only solution is to change to alternative drugs or treatment.

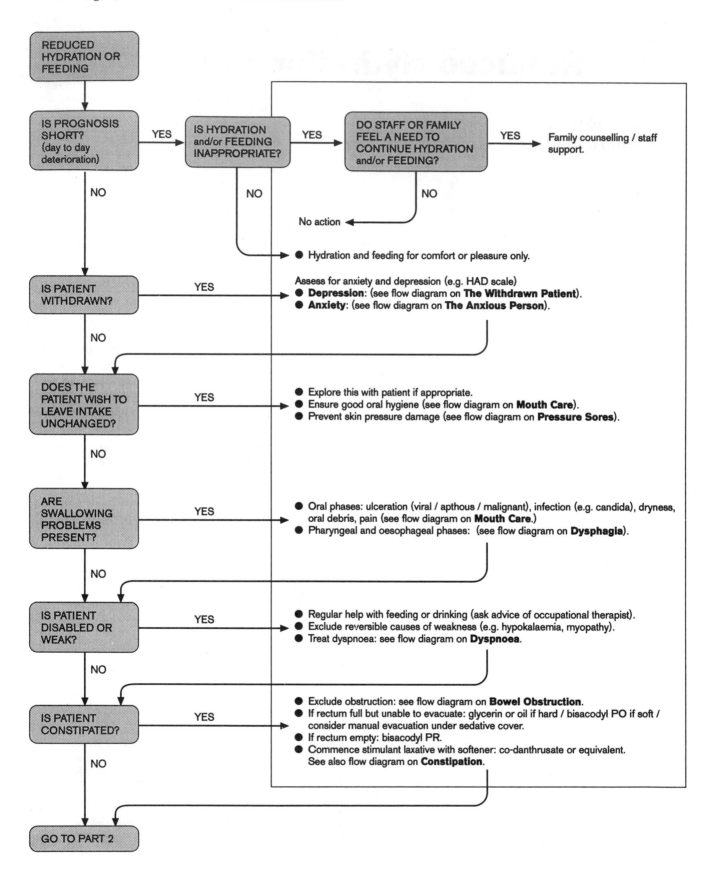

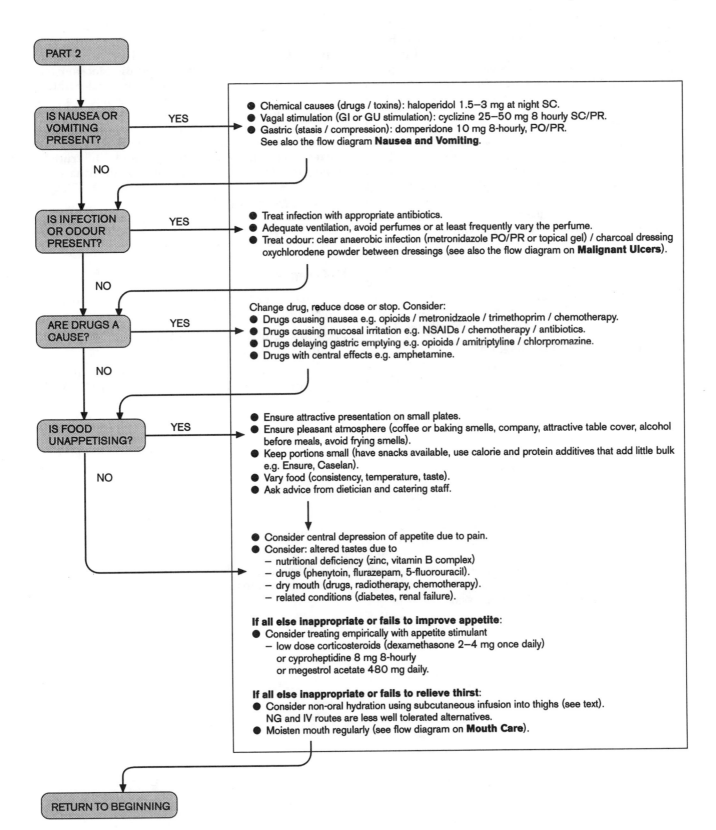

PART 2

IS NAUSEA OR VOMITING PRESENT? — YES →
- Chemical causes (drugs / toxins): haloperidol 1.5–3 mg at night SC.
- Vagal stimulation (GI or GU stimulation): cyclizine 25–50 mg 8 hourly SC/PR.
- Gastric (stasis / compression): domperidone 10 mg 8-hourly, PO/PR.
  See also the flow diagram **Nausea and Vomiting**.

NO ↓

IS INFECTION OR ODOUR PRESENT? — YES →
- Treat infection with appropriate antibiotics.
- Adequate ventilation, avoid perfumes or at least frequently vary the perfume.
- Treat odour: clear anaerobic infection (metronidazole PO/PR or topical gel) / charcoal dressing oxychlorodene powder between dressings (see also the flow diagram on **Malignant Ulcers**).

NO ↓

ARE DRUGS A CAUSE? — YES →
Change drug, reduce dose or stop. Consider:
- Drugs causing nausea e.g. opioids / metronidzaole / trimethoprim / chemotherapy.
- Drugs causing mucosal irritation e.g. NSAIDs / chemotherapy / antibiotics.
- Drugs delaying gastric emptying e.g. opioids / amitriptyline / chlorpromazine.
- Drugs with central effects e.g. amphetamine.

NO ↓

IS FOOD UNAPPETISING? — YES →
- Ensure attractive presentation on small plates.
- Ensure pleasant atmosphere (coffee or baking smells, company, attractive table cover, alcohol before meals, avoid frying smells).
- Keep portions small (have snacks available, use calorie and protein additives that add little bulk e.g. Ensure, Caselan).
- Vary food (consistency, temperature, taste).
- Ask advice from dietician and catering staff.

NO

- Consider central depression of appetite due to pain.
- Consider: altered tastes due to
  – nutritional deficiency (zinc, vitamin B complex)
  – drugs (phenytoin, flurazepam, 5-fluorouracil).
  – dry mouth (drugs, radiotherapy, chemotherapy).
  – related conditions (diabetes, renal failure).

If all else inappropriate or fails to improve appetite:
- Consider treating empirically with appetite stimulant
  – low dose corticosteroids (dexamethasone 2–4 mg once daily)
    or cyproheptidine 8 mg 8-hourly
    or megestrol acetate 480 mg daily.

If all else inappropriate or fails to relieve thirst:
- Consider non-oral hydration using subcutaneous infusion into thighs (see text).
  NG and IV routes are less well tolerated alternatives.
- Moisten mouth regularly (see flow diagram on **Mouth Care**).

RETURN TO BEGINNING

Unappetising food and drink are a common cause of reduced appetite. It is still common to find alcohol being dispensed from calibrated plastic pots, instead of from bottle to glass as part of a social occasion. Small helpings of attractively presented food are more likely to be eaten than large amorphous masses. A dietician is invaluable in advising on how to vary food and drink taste and consistency while maintaining a reasonable level of calorie and protein intake.[2] Other causes of appetite suppression are pain and reduced enjoyment due to altered taste. Taste changes are well recognised in cancer,[3] although their exact cause is often unclear. Some patients are deficient in zinc or one of the vitamin B complexes, while others are on drugs known to cause taste changes (e.g. phenytoin), or have a dry mouth due to treatment.

If no cause can be found: It is common to fail to find an easily reversible cause of reduced appetite for food or drink. Here patients may be helped by the empirical use of appetite stimulants,[4] such as low dose corticosteroids, cyproheptidine or megestrol acetate. Low dose dexamethasone (4 mg once daily) is most commonly used.

Non-oral hyddration and feeding: Enteral hydration and feeding (e.g. through a gastrostomy) is used in some patients with swallowing problems (see the flow diagram on *Dysphagia*). Intravenous feeding has been used prior to surgery or chemotherapy, but has little place in palliative care. In contrast, parenteral hydration is accepted practice in treating hypercalcaemia and severe gastric outflow obstruction. A third indication is repeated vomiting from other causes, causing rapid dehydration. It has been suggested that hydration is also appropriate for some patients with a hyperactive confusional state, especially those on opioids[5] (see the flow diagram on *Confusional States*). Whilst the intravenous route is often the first to be considered, the subcutaneous route is often simpler and better tolerated.[5,6] Normal (0.9%) saline or 5% glucose can be given into the anterior thigh through a narrow gauge intravenous plastic cannula inserted subcutaneously. Hyaluronidase is unnecessary,[6] and in our experience rates of up to 1 litre every 12 hours into each thigh are possible.

It must be noted that parenteral hydration for rapid fluid loss occurring over days is quite distinct from chronic and gentle hydration that occurs over a longer time in the final stages of a patient's life. In the absence of a hyperactive confusional state, hydration is neither appropriate nor necessary. The belief that all patients must be hydrated is incorrect, but so is the belief that no patients in the terminal stages should be hydrated. The truth is that some patients require hydration in some situations.

Acknowledgement

We are grateful to Sarah Fitton, Nursing Sister, St. Oswald's Hospice, for her useful help and advice.

References

1. Regnard CFB. Dysphagia. In: Balliere's Clinical *Oncology*, 1987, Volume **1**: 327–355.

2. Shaw C. Nutritional aspects of advanced cancer. *Palliative Medicine* 1992; **6**: 105–110.

3. De Wys WD and Walters K. Abnormalities of taste sensation in cancer patients. *Cancer*, 1975; **36**: 1888–1896.

4. Bruera E and Fainsinger RL. Clinical management of cachexia and anorexia. In: Doyle D, Hanks G and MacDonald N., eds. *Oxford Textbook of Palliative Medicine*. Oxford: Oxford University Press, 1993. pp. 330–337.

5. Fainsinger R and Bruera E. The management of dehydration in terminally ill patients. *J Pall Care*, 1994; 10: 55–59.

6. Constans T, Dutertre J and Froge E. Hypodermoclysis in dehydrated elderly patients: local effects with and without hyaluronidase. *J Pall Care*, 1991; **7**: 10–12.

⑧ Bowel Obstruction

Claud Regnard

In patients with advanced disease, bowel obstruction is most commonly associated with cancer (3%), especially with carcinoma of the colon (10%) and carcinoma of the ovary (25%). Once ileus and constipation have been excluded, obstructed patients should be considered for surgery. Such intervention, however, is not possible or appropriate for many patients with advanced disease, but their symptoms can be palliated.

Definition

Obstruction here is defined as any process preventing the movement of bowel contents distally. This may be due to extra-mural compression, intramural compression (e.g. tumour), peristaltic failure (ileus), or blockage by bowel contents (e.g. faecal impaction).

Diagnosis

Two causes to be excluded are constipation (history of constipation, constipating drugs, full rectum, abdominal masses, faeces on X-ray), and a medically treatable ileus (such as that due to anti-peristaltic drugs or hypercalcaemia). Diagnosis is mainly by history (e.g. altered bowel habit, absent flatus, vomiting, pain), observation (e.g. distension, visible peristalsis), examination (e.g. resonant percussion, succussion splash), and investigation (radiology). Vomiting is less frequent and develops later in obstructions of the distal ileum and colon, while high obstructions cause frequent vomiting at an early stage, but with little or no abdominal distension. Obstruction may be complete or partial, and may be continuous or intermittent. The more complete and continuous the obstruction, the more obvious and severe the symptoms.

Surgery

A surgical opinion should always be considered. In cancer, up to 38% of obstructions are due to a benign cause or to an unrelated second primary tumour.[1] If malignancy is the cause a simple colostomy can provide good relief, but more extensive surgery has more problems.[1] Some patients, however, are too ill, their tumour is too extensive or they do not wish further intervention. These should be treated as outlined in this algorithm.

Nausea and vomiting

Constant nausea is distressing, but often treatable. The first goal is to eliminate nausea, the second to reduce vomiting to 1–3 times a day. Occasional vomiting may continue, but patients find this is preferable to constant nausea. An antihistaminic antiemetic (e.g. cyclizine) is the first to use, adding a dopamine antagonist (e.g. haloperidol) if the nausea persists. Alternatives are to replace the cyclizine with an anticholinergic (e.g. hyoscine hydrobromide), or to consider the use of octreotide.[2,3]

Nasogastric suction

This fails to control symptoms of obstruction in at least 86% of patients.[4] It therefore has a limited place in palliative care:
- Complete obstructions lasting more than 10 days result in spread of bacterial colonisation from the colon into the small bowel. This produces malodorous, or 'faeculant' vomiting, and can be sufficiently distressing for the patient to consider a nasogastric (NG) tube.
- True faecal vomiting is due to an gastro-colic fistula and may also warrant NG suction.
- Gastric outflow obstructions in the duodenum or proximal jejunum cause forceful, repeated vomiting with rapid dehydration. H_2 blockers may have a role in reducing the volume of gastric secretion.
- Floppy stomach syndrome (see the flow diagram on *Nausea and Vomiting*).

Hydration

Distal obstructions (rectum, colon, ileum) still allow sufficient mucosal surface area for fluid absorption to prevent symptomatic dehydration. More proximal obstructions may cause mild symptoms such as a dry mouth (increased with cyclizine or hyoscine hydrobromide), which can be treated by frequent mouth care. Obstructions

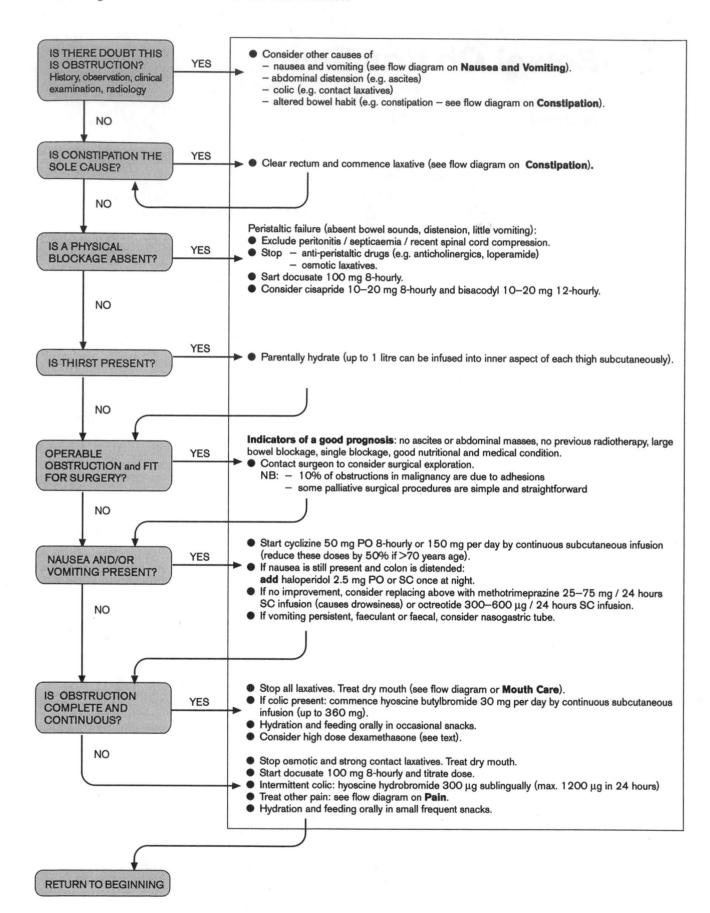

IS THERE DOUBT THIS IS OBSTRUCTION?
History, observation, clinical examination, radiology

YES

● Consider other causes of
  – nausea and vomiting (see flow diagram on **Nausea and Vomiting**).
  – abdominal distension (e.g. ascites)
  – colic (e.g. contact laxatives)
  – altered bowel habit (e.g. constipation – see flow diagram on **Constipation**).

NO

IS CONSTIPATION THE SOLE CAUSE?

YES

● Clear rectum and commence laxative (see flow diagram on **Constipation**).

NO

IS A PHYSICAL BLOCKAGE ABSENT?

YES

Peristaltic failure (absent bowel sounds, distension, little vomiting):
● Exclude peritonitis / septicaemia / recent spinal cord compression.
● Stop – anti-peristaltic drugs (e.g. anticholinergics, loperamide)
        – osmotic laxatives.
● Sart docusate 100 mg 8-hourly.
● Consider cisapride 10–20 mg 8-hourly and bisacodyl 10–20 mg 12-hourly.

NO

IS THIRST PRESENT?

YES

● Parentally hydrate (up to 1 litre can be infused into inner aspect of each thigh subcutaneously).

NO

OPERABLE OBSTRUCTION and FIT FOR SURGERY?

YES

Indicators of a good prognosis: no ascites or abdominal masses, no previous radiotherapy, large bowel blockage, single blockage, good nutritional and medical condition.
● Contact surgeon to consider surgical exploration.
  NB: – 10% of obstructions in malignancy are due to adhesions
       – some palliative surgical procedures are simple and straightforward

NO

NAUSEA AND/OR VOMITING PRESENT?

YES

● Start cyclizine 50 mg PO 8-hourly or 150 mg per day by continuous subcutaneous infusion (reduce these doses by 50% if >70 years age).
● If nausea is still present and colon is distended:
  add haloperidol 2.5 mg PO or SC once at night.
● If no improvement, consider replacing above with methotrimeprazine 25–75 mg / 24 hours SC infusion (causes drowsiness) or octreotide 300–600 µg / 24 hours SC infusion.
● If vomiting persistent, faeculant or faecal, consider nasogastric tube.

NO

IS OBSTRUCTION COMPLETE AND CONTINUOUS?

YES

● Stop all laxatives. Treat dry mouth (see flow diagram or **Mouth Care**).
● If colic present: commence hyoscine butylbromide 30 mg per day by continuous subcutaneous infusion (up to 360 mg).
● Hydration and feeding orally in occasional snacks.
● Consider high dose dexamethasone (see text).

NO

● Stop osmotic and strong contact laxatives. Treat dry mouth.
● Start docusate 100 mg 8-hourly and titrate dose.
● Intermittent colic: hyoscine hydrobromide 300 µg sublingually (max. 1200 µg in 24 hours)
● Treat other pain: see flow diagram on **Pain**.
● Hydration and feeding orally in small frequent snacks.

RETURN TO BEGINNING

proximal to the mid-jejunum may require parenteral fluids to treat symptomatic dehydration, particularly thirst. See the comments on hydration in the flow diagram on *Reduced Hydration and Feeding*.

Feeding

Patients with partial obstructions may manage small frequent snacks of low-fibre foods. Enteral feeding may be appropriate with proximal obstructions of the pharynx or oesophagus (see the flow diagram on *Dysphagia*), but parenteral nutrition is rarely needed unless as part of other treatment (e.g. surgery). Patients with complete obstructions should still be allowed to enjoy snacks as often as they wish. As a patient deteriorates the aim of feeding is for pleasure, not survival. Families and staff need to understand this as much as the patient.

Partial compared with complete obstruction

The balance in controlling symptoms in partial obstruction lies in treating colic without precipitating constipation or ileus which could create a complete obstruction. An irreversibly complete obstruction is thus usually easier to manage, since colic can be treated safely by producing a drug-induced ileus. The usefulness of corticosteroids in reducing obstruction exacerbated by peri-tumour inflammation is still unclear.

Survival

Patients managed in this way have been shown to survive for a mean of 3.7 months, with some surviving for more than 10 months, a result comparable to survival after surgery for malignant obstruction.[1]

References

1. Baines M. The pathophysiology and management of malignant intestinal obstruction. In: Doyle D, Hanks G and MacDonald N., eds. *Oxford Textbook of Palliative Medicine*. Oxford: Oxford University Press, 1993; pp. 311–316.

2. Riley J and Fallon MT. Octreotide in terminal malignant obstruction of the gastrointestinal tract. *Eur J Pall Care* 1994; **1**: 23–25.

3. Mercadante S and Maddaloni S. Octreotide in the management of inoperable gastrointestinal obstruction in terminal cancer patients. *J Pain Symp Manag* 1992; **7**: 496–498.

4. Bizer LS, Liebling RW, Delany HM and Gliedman ML. Small bowel obstruction. *Surgery* 1981; **89**: 407–413.

⑨ The Control of Diarrhoea

Claud Regnard
Kathryn Mannix

Diarrhoea is defined here as a loose or fluid stool, usually (but not invariably) accompanied by increased frequency of defecation in patients with advanced disease. This flow diagram looks at decisions required to diagnose the cause, and briefly discusses some approaches to treatment.

A loose or frequent stool is an added insult to the patient with advanced disease, especially if accompanied by perianal soreness, faecal incontinence, dehydration or abdominal pain.

Dehydration

If severe, diarrhoea can cause profound fluid and electrolyte loss (particularly potassium and bicarbonate). Causes of diarrhoea most likely to produce dehydration are infection and tumours producing vasoactive intestinal peptide (VIPomas). Clinical dehydration should be treated promptly. Enteral hydration (oral or nasogastric) should be with the WHO oral rehydration formula (for each litre: 3.5 g NaCl, 2.5 g NaHCO3, 1.5 g KCl, 20 g glucose). If the intravenous route is required, Ringer lactate solution can be used.[1]

Diagnosis of cause

Causes of intermittent diarrhoea should be considered. Constipation can produce overflow diarrhoea (see the flow diagram on *Constipation*), and partial bowel obstruction can cause episodes of diarrhoea. Gastrointestinal infection can cause diarrhoea, but repeated episodes suggest persistent infection – this can become chronic in immunocompromised patients such as those with AIDS. Carcinoid syndrome is an uncommon cause of profuse, intermittent diarrhoea. High osmotic loads to the small bowel can occur with nasogastric feeding or gastric dumping, resulting in intermittent diarrhoea.

The colour of stools may be an indication. Dark or black stools suggest bleeding from the upper gastro-intestinal tract. Steatorrhoea (a high fat content of stool) can cause diarrhoea, usually with pale stools that float and have an offensive odour. Causes of fat malabsorption include: reduced pancreatic lipases and bicarbonate due to pancreatic carcinoma or cystic fibrosis; reduced bile acids (needed to form lipid micelles prior to absorption) due to obstructive jaundice; reduced small bowel pH (resulting in reduced lipid micelle formation) due to reduced pancreatic bicarbonate (pancreatic carcinoma) or excess gastric acid production (Zollinger-Ellison syndrome); and lastly, reduced bile salt absorption (causing irritation of the colon) due to intestinal resection. Mixed melaena and steatorrhoea can occasionally produce a 'silver' stool.

Previous surgery can cause diarrhoea: gastrectomy (dumping syndrome); ileal resection (bile irritation of colon); blind loops (bacterial overgrowth); and anterior resection (mucous discharge).

Stool contents other than faeces may indicate the cause. Clear fluid in low volume may be mucus from the colon (total bowel obstruction), rectum (surgically formed rectal stump) or from a mucus secreting rectal or colonic tumour. A larger volume may be urine from a vesicocolic or vesicorectal fistula – this can be confirmed by the instillation of methylene blue into the bladder. Volumes greater than 1 litre per 24 hours suggest excessive bowel mucosal secretion (infection, VIPoma, carcinoid). Blood or offensive discharge in the stool suggests a fungating rectal or colonic carcinoma, infection (especially shigella or salmonella), or mucosal inflammation of the rectum or colon (nonsteroidal anti-inflammatory drugs,[2] radiotherapy).

Exclude: drugs (laxatives, magnesium antacids, antibiotics, β-blockers, diuretics); infection (stool culture is required if the diarrhoea persists for more than 5 days or contacts are affected); a gastrocolic fistula; irritable colon; recent radiotherapy to the lower spine or pelvis; and anxiety or fear.

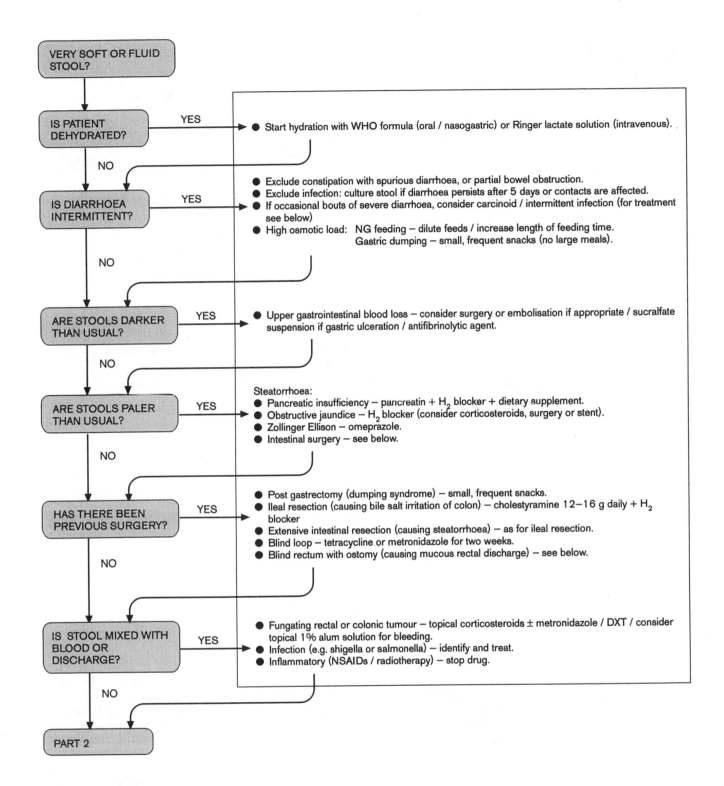

VERY SOFT OR FLUID STOOL?

IS PATIENT DEHYDRATED? — YES →
- Start hydration with WHO formula (oral / nasogastric) or Ringer lactate solution (intravenous).

NO

IS DIARRHOEA INTERMITTENT? — YES →
- Exclude constipation with spurious diarrhoea, or partial bowel obstruction.
- Exclude infection: culture stool if diarrhoea persists after 5 days or contacts are affected.
- If occasional bouts of severe diarrhoea, consider carcinoid / intermittent infection (for treatment see below)
- High osmotic load: NG feeding – dilute feeds / increase length of feeding time.
                                      Gastric dumping – small, frequent snacks (no large meals).

NO

ARE STOOLS DARKER THAN USUAL? — YES →
- Upper gastrointestinal blood loss – consider surgery or embolisation if appropriate / sucralfate suspension if gastric ulceration / antifibrinolytic agent.

NO

ARE STOOLS PALER THAN USUAL? — YES →
Steatorrhoea:
- Pancreatic insufficiency – pancreatin + H_2 blocker + dietary supplement.
- Obstructive jaundice – H_2 blocker (consider corticosteroids, surgery or stent).
- Zollinger Ellison – omeprazole.
- Intestinal surgery – see below.

NO

HAS THERE BEEN PREVIOUS SURGERY? — YES →
- Post gastrectomy (dumping syndrome) – small, frequent snacks.
- Ileal resection (causing bile salt irritation of colon) – cholestyramine 12–16 g daily + H_2 blocker
- Extensive intestinal resection (causing steatorrhoea) – as for ileal resection.
- Blind loop – tetracycline or metronidazole for two weeks.
- Blind rectum with ostomy (causing mucous rectal discharge) – see below.

NO

IS STOOL MIXED WITH BLOOD OR DISCHARGE? — YES →
- Fungating rectal or colonic tumour – topical corticosteroids ± metronidazole / DXT / consider topical 1% alum solution for bleeding.
- Infection (e.g. shigella or salmonella) – identify and treat.
- Inflammatory (NSAIDs / radiotherapy) – stop drug.

NO

PART 2

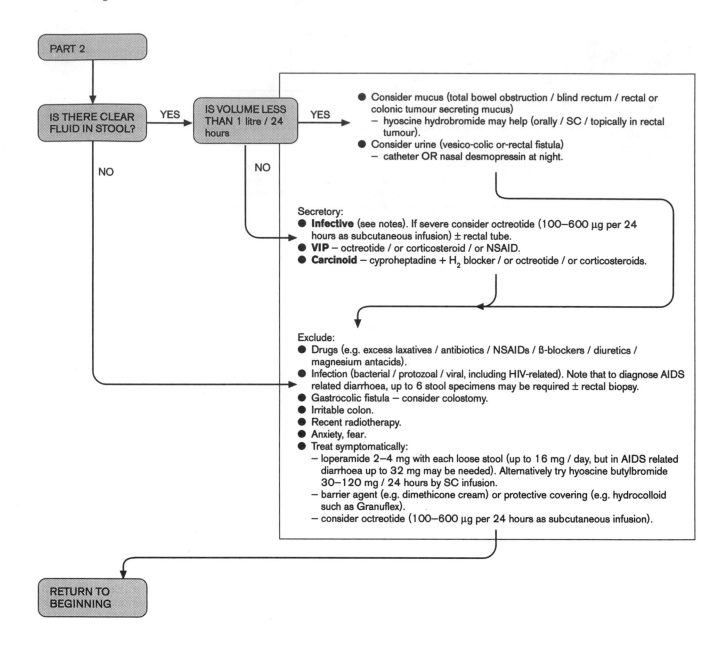

Treatment of diarrhoea

Increase water absorption: This can be done by slowing peristalsis using the peripherally acting opioid agonist, loperamide, with up to 16 mg daily. Doses of 32 mg daily or higher have been used in AIDS related diarrhoea.[3] Loperamide is preferred to drugs with anticholinergic adverse effects (e.g. atropine) or to centrally acting opioids (e.g. morphine). An alternative is hyoscine butylbromide (Buscopan) by continuous subcutaneous infusion. These drugs should be used with caution in infective diarrhoea since overgrowth of dangerous pathogens can occur.

Reduce osmotic load: Nasogastric feeds can be diluted or the rate of administration decreased. In dumping syndromes, meals should be small and frequent.

Reduce lipid malabsorption: Steatorrhoea can often be managed with drugs increasing water absorption as above.

Pancreatic insufficiency may require enzyme replacement using pancreatin tablets or capsules (lipase, protease and amylase). Duodenal pH should be increased to encourage lipid micelle formation by starting an H_2 blocker. Magnesium antacids should not be used, since they can themselves cause diarrhoea and also reduce lipid absorption, problems not shared by aluminium antacids. Dietary supplements may be required. Where obstructive jaundice is due to bile duct obstruction, high dose corticosteroids may reduce peritumour oedema and inflammation, with relief of the obstruction. Intestinal resection diminishes the release of gastrin-inhibiting hormones, resulting in increased gastrin – this increases gastric acid output which further reduces lipid micelle formation by making the duodenal content too acid. An H_2 blocker should therefore be added.

Reduce bile salt irritation: Bile salts can be sequestrated using cholestyramine.

Reduce urinary leakage: Urine from a fistula may be helped by a urethral catheter. Urine formation can be stopped at night with nasal desmopressin – this at least allows for night-time continence.[4]

Reduce mucosal secretion: Mucus production can be reduced with hyoscine hydrobromide taken systemically or applied topically. Specific remedies may be available (octreotide in VIPoma, cyproheptadine and H2 blocker or octreotide in carcinoid). With infective diarrhoea, chlorpromazine and nonsteroidal anti-inflammatory drugs have been shown to reduce secretion, although usually only at high doses that produce adverse effects. Although a rectal tube or faecal collecting device may help, it is worth considering the somatostatin analogue, octreotide. This inhibitory peptide will reduce the volume of AIDS related diarrhoea,[5, 6] and will reduce diarrhoea due to fistulae caused by malignancy.[7]

Reduce blood or discharge: Bleeding from rectal tumours can be reduced or stopped with topical 1% alum solution,[8] or sucralfate.[9] Offensive discharge may be reduced with systemic or topical metronidazole, or topical corticosteroids. Radiotherapy may help both bleeding and discharge.

Treat infection: Antimicrobial therapy is contra-indicated in most common causes of infective diarrhoea of mild to moderate severity; antibiotics may indeed worsen the situation due to selective bacterial overgrowth as with pseudomembranous colitis. Usually, only rehydration is needed. Stool microscopy and culture are essential in severe or persistent cases. In AIDS, up to six stool specimens may be required, and a wide range of organisms may be isolated or demonstrated including, protozoa (e.g. Cryptosporidium), bacteria (e.g. Salmonella, mycobacteria), viruses (e.g. cytomegalovirus) and fungi (e.g. candida).[3] When possible, treatment will be directed at a specific organism and the advice of a microbiologist is essential.

General care

The skin around the anus or a fistula needs to be protected from the excoriating effects of faecal fluid. Barrier agents such as dimethicone cream are helpful. If the skin is severely damaged, protective coverings such as hydrocolloid dressings (e.g. Granuflex) provide additional protection. In severe, persistent diarrhoea, faecal collecting devices are helpful and are obtainable from the stoma specialist.

References

1. Tomkins AM. Infections of the gastrointestinal tract. In: *Oxford Textbook of Medicine, 2nd ed.* Oxford: Oxford University Press 1987; pp. 12.164–12.178

2. Banerjee AK. Enteropathy, induced by non-steroidal anti-inflammatory drugs. *Br Med J*, 1989; **298**: 1539–40.

3. O'Neill W. AIDS related dirrhoea: a rational approach to symptomatic treatment. *Pall Med* 1992; **6**: 61–64.

4. Meadow SR and Evans JHC. Desmopressin for enuresis. *Br Med J*, 1989; **298**: 1596–7.

5. Cello JP, Basuk P *et al.* Effect of octreotide on refractory AIDS-related diarrhoea. *Ann Int Med* 1991; **115**: 705–710.

6. Mercadante S. Octreotide in treatment of AIDS-related symptoms. *Eur J Pall Care* 1994; **1**: 38–41.

7. Nubiola P, Badia JM, Martinez-Rodenas F *et al.* Treatment of 27 postoperative enterocutaneous fistulas with the long half life somatostatin analogue SMS 201–995. *Ann Surg* 1989; **210**: 56–58.

8. Paes TRF, Marsh GDJ, Morecroft JA and Hale JE. Alum solution in the control of intractable haemorrhage from advanced carcinoma. *Br J Surg*, 1986; **73**:192.

9. Regnard CFB. Control of bleeding in advanced cancer. *Lancet* 1991; **337**: 974.

10 Management of Ascites

Claud Regnard
Kathryn Mannix

Ascites is here defined as an exudate into the peritoneal space. It is most commonly due to malignancy or liver disease. It can cause symptoms such as pain, nausea, vomiting and dyspnoea. If the primary cause cannot be resolved, these symptoms are most easily resolved by removing the ascites. This can be done by mechanical means (e.g. paracentesis) or pharmacological means (e.g. diuretics). This flow diagram describes the decision steps in choosing appropriate treatment in a patient with ascites due to a process that has been diagnosed and is responding poorly, or no longer responding, to treatment.

Causes

Ascites due to malignancy is the cause of abdominal distension in 6% of patients admitted to a hospice, with the commonest primary tumours being breast, ovary, colon, stomach, pancreas and bronchus.[1]

Four types can be identified:[2]

Peripheral (the commonest type): This is caused by blockage of peritoneal lymphatics by tumour, chronic peritoneal infection or granulomatous disease. In malignancy, increased capillary permeability may also be a factor. Hypoalbuminaemia will reduce osmotic pressure and worsen the ascites. Low plasma protein is due to reduced synthesis in liver disease, and in malignancy is due to a combination of a catabolic state and increased urinary excretion of protein.

Central: This is due to intrahepatic obstruction of the portal venous and lymphatic systems by tumour or cirrhosis, or due to hepatic congestion caused by ventricular failure.

Mixed (i.e. mixed central and peripheral): This is due to conditions affecting the liver and peritoneum.

Chylous (uncommon): This is due to obstruction and leakage of retroperitoneal lymphatics.

This flow diagram assumes the primary cause of the ascites is known.

Diagnosis

Gross ascites produces a distended abdomen, sometimes with leg, perineal and lower trunk oedema. With the patient supine the abdomen is dull to percussion, although the central abdomen may be resonant; the area changes position on turning the patient – this is shifting dullness. A fluid thrill may be present. Areas dull to percussion can also be caused by abdominal tumour, ovarian cyst, hepatomegaly, pregnancy, severe bladder or gastric dilatation. The signs and symptoms of a 'squashed stomach syndrome' may be present (see the flow diagram on *Nausea and Vomiting*). In ascites due to malignancy, an abdominal bruit suggests a vascular tumour such as hepatocellular carcinoma, renal cell carcinoma or carcinoid.

Treatment

Treatment consists most effectively of removing and, if possible, preventing the return, of the ascites:

Paracentesis: Mechanical drainage of ascites provides rapid relief of troublesome symptoms. Drainage to dryness is both safe and effective when removing volumes of 5 litres or less over 24 hours.[2] Removal is better tolerated in the presence of peripheral oedema, but when this is absent, or if the amount of ascites needs drainage over several days, intravenous albumin will be required to prevent hypotension. In malignant ascites the volume is usually less than 5 litres and is safely removed slowly over 24 hours. The puncture site chosen needs to be away from scars, tumour masses, distended bowel, bladder, liver or inferior epigastric arteries. The left lower quadrant is therefore often chosen. The puncture site is infiltrated with 0.25% bupivacaine down to the peritoneum. Either a peritoneal dialysis catheter[1] or small bore suprapubic bladder drainage catheter[4] is preferable to a large-bore paracentesis trochar. Two litres are drained over the first hour for comfort, followed by drainage to dryness over the following 12 hours. The tube can then be removed and the puncture site covered by a colostomy bag for a few days while the puncture closes. Occasionally, viscous ascites is encountered. The authors have encountered success in removing mucinous ascites through the puncture site using suction, and later by enlarging the opening to produce an artificial fistula through which the ascites could be expressed into a colostomy bag.

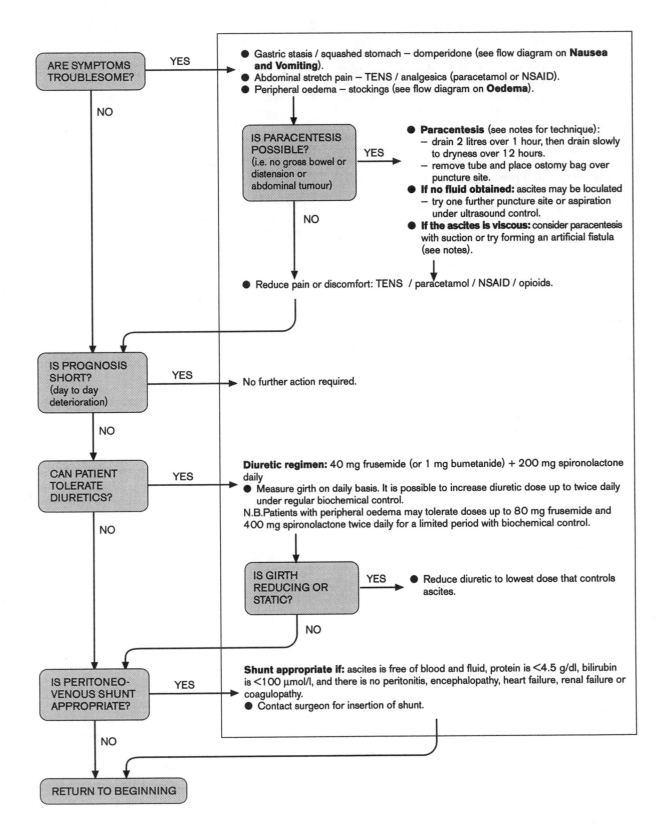

ARE SYMPTOMS TROUBLESOME? — YES →
- Gastric stasis / squashed stomach – domperidone (see flow diagram on **Nausea and Vomiting**).
- Abdominal stretch pain – TENS / analgesics (paracetamol or NSAID).
- Peripheral oedema – stockings (see flow diagram on **Oedema**).

IS PARACENTESIS POSSIBLE? (i.e. no gross bowel or distension or abdominal tumour) — YES →
- **Paracentesis** (see notes for technique):
  – drain 2 litres over 1 hour, then drain slowly to dryness over 12 hours.
  – remove tube and place ostomy bag over puncture site.
- **If no fluid obtained:** ascites may be loculated
  – try one further puncture site or aspiration under ultrasound control.
- **If the ascites is viscous:** consider paracentesis with suction or try forming an artificial fistula (see notes).

NO

- Reduce pain or discomfort: TENS / paracetamol / NSAID / opioids.

ARE SYMPTOMS TROUBLESOME? NO ↓

IS PROGNOSIS SHORT? (day to day deterioration) — YES → No further action required.

NO

CAN PATIENT TOLERATE DIURETICS? — YES →
Diuretic regimen: 40 mg frusemide (or 1 mg bumetanide) + 200 mg spironolactone daily
- Measure girth on daily basis. It is possible to increase diuretic dose up to twice daily under regular biochemical control.
N.B. Patients with peripheral oedema may tolerate doses up to 80 mg frusemide and 400 mg spironolactone twice daily for a limited period with biochemical control.

NO

IS GIRTH REDUCING OR STATIC? — YES →
- Reduce diuretic to lowest dose that controls ascites.

NO

IS PERITONEO-VENOUS SHUNT APPROPRIATE? — YES →
Shunt appropriate if: ascites is free of blood and fluid, protein is <4.5 g/dl, bilirubin is <100 μmol/l, and there is no peritonitis, encephalopathy, heart failure, renal failure or coagulopathy.
- Contact surgeon for insertion of shunt.

NO

RETURN TO BEGINNING

Diuretics: Ascites of the peripheral and mixed types appears to be associated with increased renin activity and sodium retention which is the logic for using spironolactone.[5] This is usually combined with a loop diuretic such as frusemide or bumetanide.[1] Some patients can only tolerate low doses, but patients with peripheral oedema may tolerate higher doses.[6] Patients should be monitored regularly for electrolyte disturbances.

Peritoneovenous shunt: This should be considered with recurrent ascites not controlled by diuretics. Insertion of a shunt is a 30–60 minute procedure which can be carried out under a local anaesthetic and causes fewer problems than for ascites due to non-malignant liver disease.[7] In malignant disease, although the shunt drains fluid from the peritoneal space to a neck vein, there is no evidence of increased metastatic disease.[8] In non-malignant ascites, a shunt can give good palliation, but blockage occurs sooner in malignant ascites.[2]

References

1. Twycross RG and Lack SA. Ascites, In: *Control of Alimentary Symptoms in Far Advanced Cancer.* Edinburgh: Churchill Livingstone, 1986; pp. 282–299.

2. Bain VG and Minuk GY. Jaundice, ascites and hepatic encephalopathy. In: Doyle D, Hanks G and MacDonald N., eds. *Oxford Textbook of Palliative Medicine.* Oxford: Oxford University Press, 1993; pp 342–348.

3. Editorial. Diuretics or paracentesis for ascites? *Lancet*, 1988; **ii**: 775–776.

4. Mansi JL and Hanks GW. Drainage of malignant effusions. *Lancet*, 1989; **ii**: 43.

5. Greenway B, Johnson PJ and Williams R. Control of malignant ascites with spironolactone. *Br J Surg*, 1982; **69**: 441–442.

6. Pockros PJ and Reynolds TB. Rapid diuresis in patients with ascites from chronic liver disease: the importance of peripheral oedema. *Gastroenterology*, 1986; **90**: 1827–1833.

7. Rubenstein D, McInnes I and Dudley F. Morbidity and mortality after peritoneovenous shunt surgery for refractory ascites. *Gut*, 1985; **26**: 1070–1073.

8. Tarin D, Price JE, Kettlewell MGW, et al. Clinicopathological observations on metastases in man studied in patients with peritoneovenous shunts. *Br Med J*, 1984; **288**: 749–751.

11 Urinary Problems

Claud Regnard
Kathryn Mannix

Problems related to the urinary system may accompany many diseases or be their cause. This flow diagram deals with the management of common urinary symptoms and with some special urinary problems associated with advanced disease.

Altered appearance of urine

A crystal clear urine of normal colour and negative for nitrites and leukocyte esterase on ward testing, can be considered free of infection, making culture unnecessary in most cases.[1] Any cloudiness may be due to infection or excess protein. Cloudiness suggests infection if one or more of the following symptoms is present: positive testing for nitrites, dysuria, frequency, incontinence, strong smelling urine, pyrexia, unilateral loin pain or confusion. If the patient has a normal genitourinary tract and is female a single dose of an appropriate antibiotic is acceptable.[2] If symptoms persist or the patient is male the urine should be cultured and a single dose of the recommended antibiotic should be given. If symptoms still persist or the genitourinary tract is abnormal (e.g. tumour involvement or catheter in place), the antibiotic recommended by culture should be given for two weeks or longer if pyelonephritis is present. Patients with urethral catheters invariably have a colonised urine and treatment is only necessary in the presence of pyrexia, or pain from the urethra or bladder.

Colour change may be due to haematuria or excreted products. For microscopic haematuria or excreted products no action is necessary and patients should be reassured. Heavy bleeding producing clots or anaemia should be treated with a 1% solution of alum.[3] This can be instilled and left for 15 minutes, or can be used as an irrigating solution through a three way catheter if the bleeding is more troublesome. Patients with persistent bleeding should be considered for palliative radiotherapy to bladder, prostate or kidney, depending on the source of bleeding. Arterial embolisation may also be helpful.

Pain

This has several causes, each indicated by their site:

Urethral pain (usually felt at the tip of the urethra) is usually due to direct irritation or referred pain from the trigone. Instilling 20 ml 0.25% bupivacaine into the bladder for 15 minutes gives good relief for 8–12 hours. If a catheter is in place it may help to reduce the balloon volume, or to consider intermittent catheterisation (see below).

Central, lower abdominal pain can be caused by bladder colic and occasionally can be continuous. Urinary retention must be excluded. In addition to the treatments above, anticholinergic drugs such as imipramine or hyoscine butylbromide (Buscopan) can be helpful. Hyoscine butylbromide can be given by a continuous subcutaneous infusion of 30–180 mg in 24 hours with few central effects, but with an inhibiting action on bowel motility.

Groin pain may be due to ureteric colic and can also be continuous on occasions. When severe, ureteric colic is most effectively treated with diclofenac IM or PR, although hyoscine butylbromide IV or SC can be equally effective but will not last as long. It is often inappropriate to try to reverse ureteric obstructions in advanced cancer, but some procedures are worth considering in patients with smaller tumour loads. Obstructions can be relieved with ureteric stents inserted at cystoscopy, while obstructions due to peritumour oedema may be eased by high dose corticosteroids (18–24 mg dexamethasone starting dose). A percutaneous nephrostomy (ideally done under ultrasound control) can be helpful as a temporary measure if more radical tumour control is planned.

Renal pain due to damage by tumour, infection or haemorrhage will usually require strong opioids with the addition of a non-steroidal anti-inflammatory drug (Sulindac is less likely than other NSAIDs to cause further renal impairment). Radiotherapy can palliate a painful renal tumour, if there is a functioning kidney on the other side.

Urinary incontinence

This can be due to several causes:

Urinary fistulae are easily missed, but can be readily identified by instilling methylene blue into the bladder through a temporary catheter. Incontinence due to a fistula can be partly eased by measures such as pads, frequent voiding and continuous catheterisation. A vesico-vaginal fistula can be helped with a vaginal prosthesis made of silicone which incorporates a catheter using the technique suggested by Green and Phillips.[4] Urinary diversion is not usually appropriate. If all else fails, dry nights can be provided by using nasal desmopressin (10–40 μg) at bedtime.[5] When desmopressin is given, no fluids are given after 6 pm and it is important to make sure that patients have a daytime output of at least 500 ml.

Total urethral incontinence: This is usually due to tumour invasion, and requires an indwelling catheter.[6]

Overflow due to outflow obstruction should always be considered and treated appropriately (see urethral obstruction below).

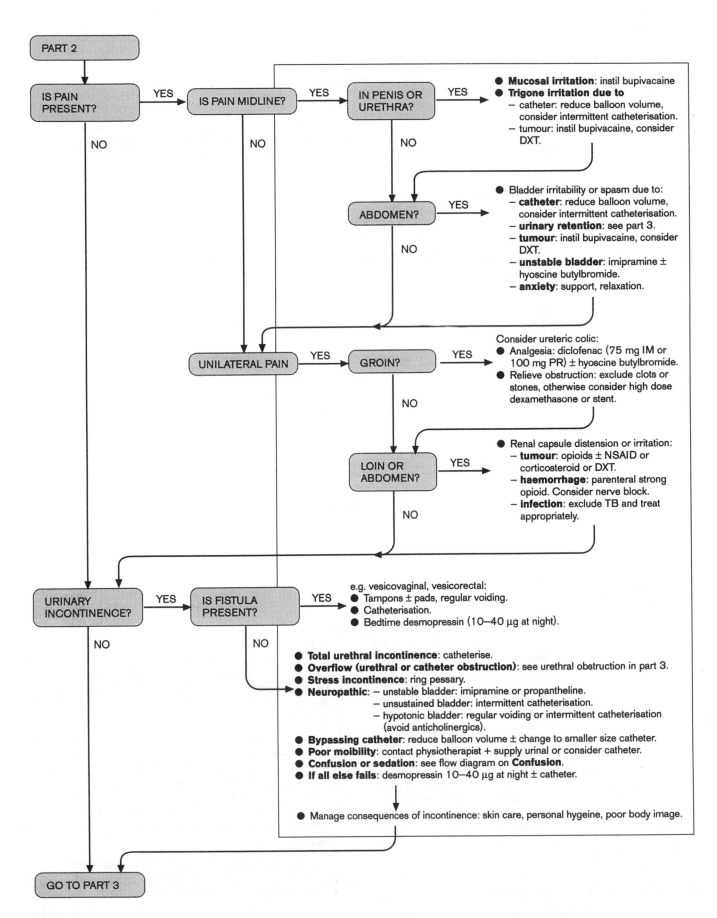

PART 2

IS PAIN PRESENT? — YES → IS PAIN MIDLINE? — YES → IN PENIS OR URETHRA? — YES →
- **Mucosal irritation**: instil bupivacaine
- **Trigone irritation due to**
  - catheter: reduce balloon volume, consider intermittent catheterisation.
  - tumour: instil bupivacaine, consider DXT.

IN PENIS OR URETHRA? — NO → ABDOMEN? — YES →
- Bladder irritability or spasm due to:
  - **catheter**: reduce balloon volume, consider intermittent catheterisation.
  - **urinary retention**: see part 3.
  - **tumour**: instil bupivacaine, consider DXT.
  - **unstable bladder**: imipramine ± hyoscine butylbromide.
  - **anxiety**: support, relaxation.

IS PAIN MIDLINE? — NO → UNILATERAL PAIN — YES → GROIN? — YES →
Consider ureteric colic:
- Analgesia: diclofenac (75 mg IM or 100 mg PR) ± hyoscine butylbromide.
- Relieve obstruction: exclude clots or stones, otherwise consider high dose dexamethasone or stent.

GROIN? — NO → LOIN OR ABDOMEN? — YES →
- Renal capsule distension or irritation:
  - **tumour**: opioids ± NSAID or corticosteroid or DXT.
  - **haemorrhage**: parenteral strong opioid. Consider nerve block.
  - **infection**: exclude TB and treat appropriately.

IS PAIN PRESENT? — NO

URINARY INCONTINENCE? — YES → IS FISTULA PRESENT? — YES →
e.g. vesicovaginal, vesicorectal:
- Tampons ± pads, regular voiding.
- Catheterisation.
- Bedtime desmopressin (10–40 µg at night).

IS FISTULA PRESENT? — NO →
- **Total urethral incontinence**: catheterise.
- **Overflow (urethral or catheter obstruction)**: see urethral obstruction in part 3.
- **Stress incontinence**: ring pessary.
- **Neuropathic**: – unstable bladder: imipramine or propantheline.
  – unsustained bladder: intermittent catheterisation.
  – hypotonic bladder: regular voiding or intermittent catheterisation (avoid anticholinergics).
- **Bypassing catheter**: reduce balloon volume ± change to smaller size catheter.
- **Poor moibility**: contact physiotherapist + supply urinal or consider catheter.
- **Confusion or sedation**: see flow diagram on **Confusion**.
- **If all else fails**: desmopressin 10–40 µg at night ± catheter.

- Manage consequences of incontinence: skin care, personal hygeine, poor body image.

URINARY INCONTINENCE? — NO

GO TO PART 3

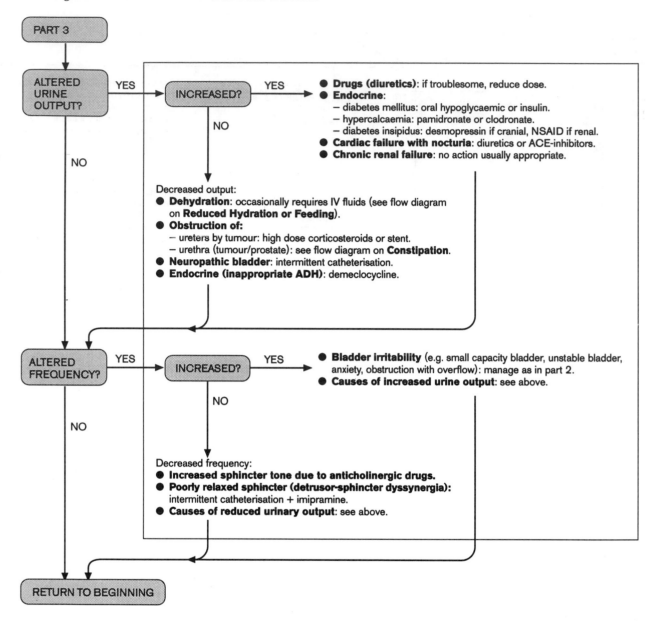

PART 3

ALTERED URINE OUTPUT? — YES → **INCREASED?** — YES →
- **Drugs (diuretics)**: if troublesome, reduce dose.
- **Endocrine**:
  – diabetes mellitus: oral hypoglycaemic or insulin.
  – hypercalcaemia: pamidronate or clodronate.
  – diabetes insipidus: desmopressin if cranial, NSAID if renal.
- **Cardiac failure with nocturia**: diuretics or ACE-inhibitors.
- **Chronic renal failure**: no action usually appropriate.

NO ↓

Decreased output:
- **Dehydration**: occasionally requires IV fluids (see flow diagram on **Reduced Hydration or Feeding**).
- **Obstruction of**:
  – ureters by tumour: high dose corticosteroids or stent.
  – urethra (tumour/prostate): see flow diagram on **Constipation**.
- **Neuropathic bladder**: intermittent catheterisation.
- **Endocrine (inappropriate ADH)**: demeclocycline.

ALTERED FREQUENCY? — YES → **INCREASED?** — YES →
- **Bladder irritability** (e.g. small capacity bladder, unstable bladder, anxiety, obstruction with overflow): manage as in part 2.
- **Causes of increased urine output**: see above.

NO ↓

Decreased frequency:
- **Increased sphincter tone due to anticholinergic drugs.**
- **Poorly relaxed sphincter (detrusor-sphincter dyssynergia)**: intermittent catheterisation + imipramine.
- **Causes of reduced urinary output**: see above.

RETURN TO BEGINNING

Stress incontinence in women may respond to a ring pessary if an anterior vaginal prolapse is present, but usually pelvic floor exercises and/or surgery are necessary if the patient is fit enough.

A hypotonic (neuropathic) bladder may develop as a result of radical pelvic surgery, spinal cord compression below T11, damage to the sacral plexus, or following an episode of outlet obstruction. Features include difficulty in initiating micturition, an intermittent stream, incomplete emptying, stress incontinence, persistent dribbling incontinence, and recurrent infections. Intermittent catheterisation is the treatment of choice. The technique is underused and yet is safe, effective and suitable for both men and women. At least four times a day patients should use the following technique[7] during which sterility is *not* necessary, only cleanliness:

(a) wash the hands
(b) wash the skin around the urethra

(c) insert a 10FG catheter (only men require a lubricant) until urine flows
(d) once the urine has stopped gently rotate the catheter and, if no more urine flows, slowly withdraw catheter
(e) rinse the catheter in tap water and leave it immersed in a 0.016% sodium hypochlorite solution (5 ml Milton No.1 in 300 ml water).

An unstable bladder (detrusor hyper-reflexia) can be produced by damage to suprasacral pathways. It can produce frequency, nocturia, urgency, urge incontinence and nocturnal enuresis. Low dose imipramine (10–20 mg) can be very helpful, although a few patients require higher doses (100 mg or more) or a more potent anticholinergic drug such as propantheline (15–30 mg, 8-hourly).[8]

Unsustained bladder: Occasionally, symptoms due to an unstable bladder are worsened by anticholinergic drugs, resulting in repeated infections and persistent incontinence.

This 'unsustained' bladder is a feature of many central nervous system diseases, especially multiple sclerosis and spinal cord injury. Most patients will respond to intermittent catheterisation, and may be able to void normally after a few weeks or months. Patients with a long prognosis (years) may benefit from an implantable sacral nerve stimulator.

Bypassing catheters are usually due to large balloons (reduce them by half) or to a catheter that is too big (always use a 4 mm diameter – 12CH – size in first-time catheterisations). Other causes of incontinence include inappropriate behaviour due to confusion or excessive sedation, poor mobility and faecal impaction causing retention with overflow. These need to be treated as appropriate.

If all else fails, nightime incontinence can be managed with desmopressin as for urinary fistula (above).

Altered urinary output

Drugs and several diseases will increase urinary output over 24 hours or at night, and are treated as appropriate. Reduced output can be caused by dehydration and rarely needs treating.

Ureteric obstruction is treated as above.

Urethral obstruction will produce difficulty initiating micturition and a poor stream. Some patients with benign prostatic hypertrophy will respond to 20 mg indoramin at night (beware hypotension after the first dose), titrated by 20 mg every 2 weeks up to maximum of 40 mg twice daily. Malignant obstructions may respond to high dose corticosteroids, but are likely to require a urethral catheter – suprapubic catheters are rarely required. Blocked catheters usually need replacing – regular washouts are not recommended since they introduce infection. Obstructive symptoms also can be a feature of a hypotonic bladder and require intermittent catheterisation. If obstructive symptoms are present together with those of an unstable bladder, this may be due to detrusor-sphincter dyssynergia, which is usually due to spinal cord damage. This combination of problems usually responds to intermittent catheterisation and imipramine.

Inappropriate ADH secretion is an occasional feature of some tumours, notably bronchial carcinoma, and can respond to 600 mg demeclocycline 12-hourly, reducing to 300–450 mg 12 hourly for maintenance.

Diabetes mellitus: Treatment should be aimed at preventing thirst, polyuria and hypoglycaemia, rather than preventing future complications. Consequently strict control is unecessary.

Altered urinary frequency

Increased frequency is usually due to the causes of bladder irritability mentioned above. Reduced frequency can be due to anticholinergic drugs and any cause of reduced urinary output.

Indwelling catheters

These may be required for urinary problems mentioned above, or simply because a patient is too weak or in too much pain to move. It is best to use smaller size (4–5 mm) silicone coated catheters. Prior to insertion of catheters in males the urethra should be filled with 10 ml 2% lignocaine jelly. If given a full 5 minutes to take effect this will reduce discomfort during the procedure and allow the external sphincter to relax.[6] If a urethral catheter cannot be inserted, a suprapubic catheter can be placed using a sheath and trochar in the midline, 5 cm above the pubis, using a syringe and needle to confirm the position of the distended bladder. Microbiological contamination of urine is inevitable with an indwelling catheter, but the use of closed drainage systems and changing catheters every 3–4 weeks will reduce blockage and symptomatic infection. Taking vitamin C (1–2 g daily) or regularly drinking cranberry juice may lessen infections and blockages.

Acknowledgements

We are grateful to Prof. DE Neal, Professor of Surgery and Consultant Urological Surgeon (Newcastle-upon-Tyne), and Dr. Wendy Makin, Consultant in Palliative Medicine (St. Oswald's Hospice, Newcastle-upon-Tyne) for their advice in the original flow diagram in *Palliative Medicine*.

References

1. Flanagan PG, Rooney PG, Davies EA and Stout RW. Evaluation of four screening tests for bacteriuria in elderly people. *Lancet*, 1989; i: 1117–8.

2. Tolkoff-Rubin NE and Rubin RH. New approaches to the treatment of urinary tract infection. *Am J Med*, 1987; **82**(suppl 4A): 270–277.

3. Goel AK, Rao MS, Bhagwat AG *et al* Intravesical irrigation with alum for the control of massive bladder haemorrhage. *J Urol*, 1985; **133**: 956–7.

4. Green DE and Phillips GL. Vaginal prosthesis for control of vesicovaginal fistula. *Gynaecol Oncol*, 1986; **23**: 119–123.

5. Rittig S, Knusden B, Sorensen S *et al.* Longterm double-blind crossover study of desmopressin intranasal spray in the management of nocturnal enuresis. In: *Desmopressin in Nocturnal Enuresis*, Medow SR, ed., Sutton Coldfield: Horus Medical 1989;. pp. 43–55.

6. MacKinnon KJ and Norman RW. Genitourinary disorders in palliative medicine. In: Doyle D, Hanks G and MacDonald N., eds. *Oxford Textbook of Palliative Medicine*. Oxford: Oxford University Press, 1993; pp. 415–422.

7. Anonymous. Underused: intermittent self catheterisation. *Drug Ther Bull*, 1991; **29**: 37–39.

8. Malone L, Falder M and Budden C. Urinary incontinence, In: *Rehabilitation of the Physically Disabled Adult*, Goodwill CJ and Chamberlain MA eds., London, Croom Helm; 1988;. pp. 479–498.

12 Bleeding

Claud Regnard
Wendy Makin

Bleeding is defined here as any escape of blood from vessels due to causes related to advanced disease, but excluding surgery or trauma. The risk of major, external haemorrhage is often considerably exaggerated amongst staff. Bleeding of all types occurs in 14% of patients with advanced disease.[1] It is the cause of death in approximately 6% of patients,[2] but in these patients catastrophic, external haemorrhage is less common than internal, unseen bleeding. This flow diagram looks at ways to manage the varied sources and causes of bleeding, and indicates the decisions required.

While there are many potential sources of bleeding with several potential causes, treatment is limited to radiotherapeutic, pharmacological or physical approaches.

Radiotherapy

This should always be considered for a superficial bleeding tumour such as breast carcinoma, provided that there has been no previous irradiation. Some sites such as the vulva and perineum tolerate treatment less well, and even palliative doses can produce troublesome skin reactions in a debilitated patient. Radiotherapy achieves useful palliation in bronchial carcinoma for over 75% of patients with haemoptysis, and similarly can be used for haematuria where treatment is directed to kidney or bladder. Single treatments are possible in frail patients, although fractionated regimens may be used where the prognosis is at least weeks or months. Bleeding from oesophageal or rectal carcinomas can also be palliated with radiotherapy, but sensitivity of the remaining gastrointestinal tract and surrounding tissues restricts its wider use. Most patients will be treated by the familiar external beam technique, but some situations are amenable to brachytherapy, where the radioactive source is placed close to the tumour. Intravaginal and intrauterine sources have long been used in the treatment of gynaecological malignancies, and are still valuable in controlling bleeding from advanced disease. Applicators containing radioactive sources have been devised to treat oesophageal and bronchial carcinomas. Using intraluminal therapy, useful palliation can be given to these patients as day cases, in a single session.

Pharmacological

This involves modifying the coagulation mechanism. Coagulation can be encouraged by the use of topical agents, or enhanced by the use of systemic agents. Anticoagulation may be required when excess clotting is rapidly using up clotting factors, with the risk of bleeding.

Systemic: The antifibrinolytic tranexamic acid inhibits the breakdown of fibrin clots. It is well absorbed orally and most is excreted unchanged in the bladder. This would seem to make it ideal for bladder haemorrhage, but the experience of urologists is that its use results in very hard clots which can be difficult to remove and may produce obstruction. This is not a problem in other sites of bleeding, but adverse effects are nausea, diarrhoea, headache, pruritis, skin rash, muscle pains and thrombosis. Ethamsylate is thought to enhance platelet adhesion, an essential step in both the intrinsic and common pathways of coagulation. It is rapidly absorbed orally and most is excreted unchanged in the urine. This makes it an alternative to tranexamic acid for bladder haemorrhage. Adverse effects are nausea, headache and rash. Heparin and clotting factor replacement are used when severe disseminated intravascular coagulopathy (DIC) is being actively treated, especially when the underlying disease is also being actively treated. In advanced disease such active treatment is not usually appropriate, but the advice of a haematologist is invaluable, particularly as some cases of DIC with fibrinolysis respond to a simpler regimen of aminocaproic acid and low dose heparin.[3] Platelet transfusions can alleviate the distress of multifocal bleeding due to thrombocytopaenia, but are appropriate only if there is a reversible cause for the thrombocytopaenia. Fortunately such situations are uncommon, and even when they occur they are often in the last hours or days of life when the aim is to reduce distressing bleeding, usually using topical agents, rather than to treat the underlying cause.

Topical: Tranexamic acid has been used topically in bleeding rectal carcinoma[4] and may have topical applications elsewhere. Aluminium astringents such as alum are older and cheaper alternatives that act by stimulating the extrinsic pathway, binding to fibrin to prevent its removal and coagulating exposed proteins to form a protective layer which is not absorbed.[5] The addition of a sucrose

```
┌─────────────┐                    If there is a risk of bleeding:
│  BLEEDING?  │────── NO ──────►   ● If on warfarin: keep INR to between 1.5 and 3.
└─────────────┘                    ● Coagulation disorder: correct if appropriate and possible.
       │                           ● Erosive tumour: radiotherapy or embolisation / keep green towel and sedation to hand.
      YES
       │
┌─────────────┐                    ● If resuscitation is appropriate: obtain IV access
│ IS PATIENT  │────── YES ─────►      − start rapid infusion of 0.9% saline and cross match.
│ HYPOTENSIVE?│                       − commence Dextran 70 infusion while awaiting blood.
└─────────────┘                       Then: find bleeding source: visual / endoscopy / radiology.
       │                            ● If resuscitation inappropriate:
      NO                               − sedation: diazepam 5−30 mg IV
       │                                 (If no access give diazepam PR or midazolam 5−15 mg IM into deltoid).
       │                               − external bleeding: use green or blue towel to make appearance of blood less distressing to
       │                                 patient or relatives.
       │
       │                            ● Exclude coagulation disorder:
       │                               − low or abnormal platelets
       │                               − reduced warfarin metabolism or displaced warfarin (high INR)
       │                               − disseminated intravascular coagulopathy
       │                               − severe hepatic impairment
       │                               Treatment can be difficult − the adivce of a haematologist is essential.
       │
┌─────────────┐                    ● If vessel can be identified: apply pressure to stop flow.
│ IS BLEEDING │────── YES ─────►   ● Promote clotting: Apply sucralfate paste or calcium alginate dressing.
│   SOURCE    │                    ● Prevent rebleeding
│  EXTERNAL?  │                       − start ethamsylate PO 500 mg 6-hourly or tranexamic acid 1G 8-hourly.
└─────────────┘                       − apply sucralfate paste under totally non-adherent dressing (e.g. Mepitel) − dressing can be
       │                                left for up to 7 days, although rebleeding may require up to daily application of sucralfate
      NO                                paste.
       │                                Consider diathermy, radiotherapy or embolisation.
┌─────────────┐
│ GO TO PART 2│
└─────────────┘
```

molecule to the aluminium compound as in sucralfate, enhances protection against further injury as well as making the protective layer a thick gel. A 1% solution of alum has been used to treat severe bladder haemorrhage: published evidence describes 24–72 hours of constant irrigation at a rate of 5 ml/hour,[6] but less severe bleeding can be managed with 30 minute instillations from one to five times daily. Alum solution can also be used in other accessible sites such as rectal carcinoma[7] or breast carcinoma, but is inconvenient. A better alternative is sucralfate paste.[8] At present the simplest way to make such a paste is to disperse a one gram tablet of sucralfate with 2–3 ml of water soluble gel (e.g. KY jelly). The resulting mixture is adherent and easily applied to bleeding sites once or twice daily. Sucralfate alone is useful in bleeding caused by a gastric carcinoma[9] or post radiotherapy rectal proctitis,[10] but can also be useful in oral and oesophageal bleeding. Patients tend to prefer the suspension to the tablets. Vasoconstrictors such as adrenaline are only useful in the initial stages of bleeding control and should be accompanied by another means of controlling bleeding. Sclerosing agents such as phenol, silver nitrate and formalin act in a similar way to aluminium astringents, but should be avoided because they cause tissue damage, with pain and impaired healing.

Physical

Dressings: Haemastatic dressings (e.g. calcium alginate dressing such as Kaltostat) act as a matrix for coagulation, and also enhance the intrinsic and common coagulation pathways. Calcium alginate swells to a gel and is only slowly absorbed. Cellulose should be avoided as it inhibits epithelialisation and can cause irritation and foreign body reactions. Totally non-adherent dressings (e.g. Mepitel) can be left in place for up to 7 days with minimum disturbance to the fragile ulcer surface.

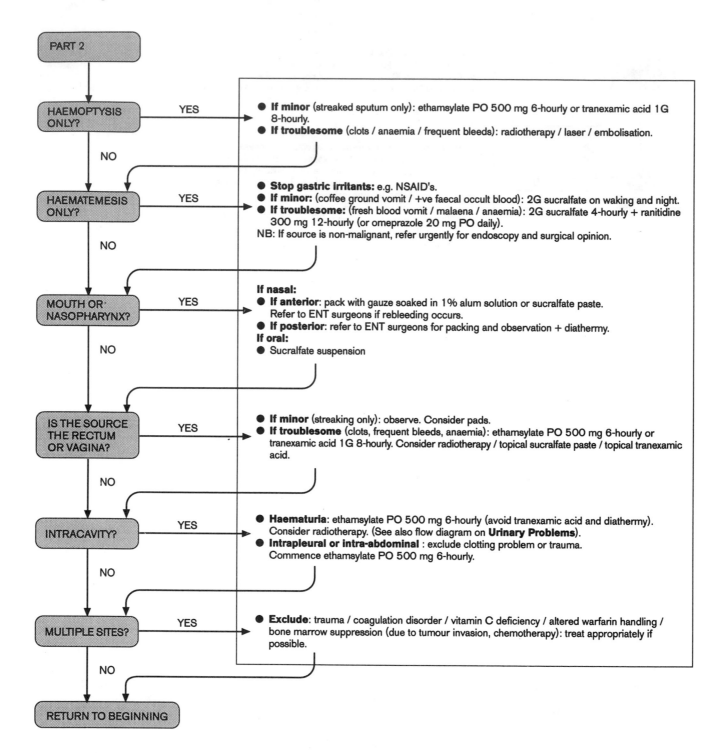

Heat and cold: bleeding lesions can be successfully treated with laser, diathermy or cryotherapy. Fungating lesions can be debulked using lasers. Lasers can also be used in any endoscopically accessible site within the bronchial tree and gastrointestinal tract, but the procedure is only available in some centres and carries a small risk of perforation. Diathermy may make haematuria worse[11] and should be avoided for bladder haemorrhage. Cryotherapy is sometimes helpful in easily accessible sites.

Embolisation is occasionally used for liver and renal malignancy and is usually performed by an interventional radiologist. Very precise tumour necrosis can be achieved, with consequent tumour shrinkage. It can be helpful in troublesome haemoptyses, and in haematuria arising from the bladder[12] or the prostate.[13] It has also been used to control bleeding from bleeding malignant ulcers.[14] It should never be used for lesions above the neck or for intraperitoneal sources. Pain and pyrexia for a few days after embolisation are the usual adverse effects.

Coping with severe, untreatable haemorrhage

Severe internal bleeding is usually from the lower gastrointestinal tract and is managed symptomatically. Pads are often sufficient, but if the blood loss is massive and a terminal event, sheets and towels can be placed in the bed to temporarily soak up the loss. The hypotension will make the patient feel cold and will be helped by warm blankets or heat pads. Although uncommon, massive haemoptysis or haematemesis are distressing because of their appearance and suddenness. If available, dark green towels or sheets mask blood effectively, and are less frightening. In any type of massive haemorrhage patients will feel frightened. Whilst some will be eased by gentle support, others will need pharmacological help. Intravenous diazepam is the most rapid and effective method. If it is felt that the risk of haermorrhage is high, it is reasonable to place a peripheral IV access cannula in the hand or arm, in case rapid IV administration is required. Alternatives are diazepam injection solution rectally or midazolam into deltoid muscle. Usually they will be absorbed and act within 5–15 minutes. Both family and staff will need support after such an experience.

References

1. Annual reports (1975–1984). St. Christopher's Hospice.

2. Carter RL. Some pathological aspects of advanced malignant disease. In: Saunders C, ed. *The Management of Terminal Malignant Disease, 3rd edition.* London: Edward Arnold, 1993.

3. Cooper DL, Sandler AB, Wilson LD and Duffy TP. Disseminated intravascular coagulation and excessive fibrinolysis in a patient with metastatic prostate cancer. *Cancer* 1992; **70**: 656–658.

4. McElligot E, Quigley C and Hanks GW. Tranexamic acid and rectal bleeding. *Lancet*, 1991; **337**: 431.

5. Hollander D and Tarnawski A. The protective and therapeutic mechanisms of sucralfate. *Scand J Gastroenterol*, 1990; **25** (suppl 173): 1–5.

6. Goel AK, Rao MS, Bhagwat *et al*. Intravesical irrigation with alum for the control of massive bladder haemorrhage. *J Urol*, 1985; **133**: 956–957.

7. Paes TRF, Marsh GDJ, Morecroft JA and Hale JE. Alum solution in the control of intractable haemorrhage from advanced rectal carcinoma. *Br J Surg*, 1986; **73**: 192.

8. Regnard CFB. Control of bleeding in advanced cancer. *Lancet*, 1991; **337**: 974.

9. Regnard CFB, Mannix K. Palliation of gastric carcinoma haemorrhage with sucralfate. *Palliative Medicine*, 1990; **4**: 329–30.

10. Kochhar R, Sharma SC. Gupta BB and Mehta SK. Rectal sucralfate in radiation proctitis. *Lancet*, 1988; i: 400.

11. Bullock N and Whitaker RH. Massive bladder haemorrhage. *Br Med J*, 1985; **291**: 1522–1523.

12. Lang EK, Deutsch JS, Goodman JR *et al*. Transcatheter embolization of hypogastric branch arteries in the management of intractable bladder haemorrhage. *J Urol* 1979; **121**: 30–36.

13. Appleton DS, Sibley GNA and Doyle PT. Internal iliac artery embolisation of bladder and prostate haemorrhage. *Br J Urol* 1988; **61**: 45–47.

14. Rankin EM, Rubens RD and Redy JF. Transcatheter embolisation to control severe bleeding in fungating breast cancer. *Eur J Surg Oncol*, 1988; **14**: 27–32.

13 Dyspnoea

Sam Ahmedzai
Claud Regnard

Dyspnoea is defined here as the subjective sensation in patients with advanced disease where the demand for oxygen is greater than the body's ability to supply oxygen. This flow diagram describes the decision processes required to manage such patients.

Our need for oxygen is constant and any actual or perceived threat to this supply is a frightening experience. This is especially so if the dyspnoea is present at rest when no respite can be found. Since dyspnoea is a subjective experience, its severity does not always correlate with pathology – the intensity should therefore be judged by the patient's expression of their distress. Consequently treatment should be both prompt and appropriate.

Basic considerations

Hypoxia of recent onset (minutes to days) often causes an agitated confusional state. Causes include major lung collapse, pneumothorax, pulmonary embolism, ventricular failure or rapidly increasing pleural effusion. Increasing the inspired oxygen concentration may help if there is still enough intact area for gas exchange. Since hypoxia is not always accompanied by central cyanosis, however, it is valuable to confirm the presence of hypoxia by measuring oxygen saturation with a bedside oximeter, although such instruments are not available in most palliative care settings.

The subjective element of dyspnoea can be eased by a variety of measures, including gentle and sure explanation, massage (especially with aromatic oils), distraction (such as music), and increased air movement across face and chest (open windows, fan). Dyspnoea developing over days or weeks can be eased by teaching the patient relaxation exercises. Some patients may be more comfortable in a soft chair and may prefer sleeping in this position. Lying on the affected side and the use of soft pillows and a bedcradle are soothing. Fitting mobility to the limits set by the dyspnoea is important, and a physiotherapist is invaluable.

Rapidly developing dyspnoea

When dyspnoea occurs in minutes or hours the following is recommended:

Acute ventricular failure is treated conventionally with loop diuretics IV, followed by an ACE inhibitor. Ventricular failure may be precipitated by a pulmonary embolus or pericardial effusion – see below.

Localised acute airways obstruction: Stridor can be caused by malignant obstruction of the airway, vocal cord paralysis due to mediastinal tumour, or laryngeal oedema due to superior vena caval obstruction (SVCO). It requires the immediate administration of high dose corticosteroid to reduce peritumour oedema: e.g. initially 24 mg IV, followed by 16 mg PO daily. If a bovine cough is present the patient should be referred urgently to the ear, nose and throat specialists to assess vocal cord function, since these patients occasionally require emergency tracheostomy. Following emergency treatment obstructed patients should always be considered for further prompt treatment (e.g. radiotherapy, stent insertion or laser[1]).

Generalised acute airways obstruction may be precipitated by infection, particularly in the presence of chronic obstructive airways disease (COAD). The chronic asthmatic may also present with multiple attacks. Bronchodilators are the mainstay of treatment and for severe attacks are best nebulised e.g. 2.5–5 mg salbutamol nebulised every 6 hours. Corticosteroids may help either orally (25–50 mg prednisolone daily, or 4–8 mg dexamethasone daily), by inhaler or nebuliser (see guidelines on management of asthma[2]), or parenterally (100–300 mg hydrocortisone daily).

Pericardial effusion: This is identified by hypotension, dyspnoea, tachycardia, a wide area of cardiac dullness, raised venous pressure and an exaggerated drop in arterial pressure on inspiration. Referral to a cardiology unit may be appropriate, but when symptoms develop rapidly the need for aspiration is urgent – this is best done through the sub-xiphisternal route under ECG monitoring, with the needle connected to one of the chest leads.

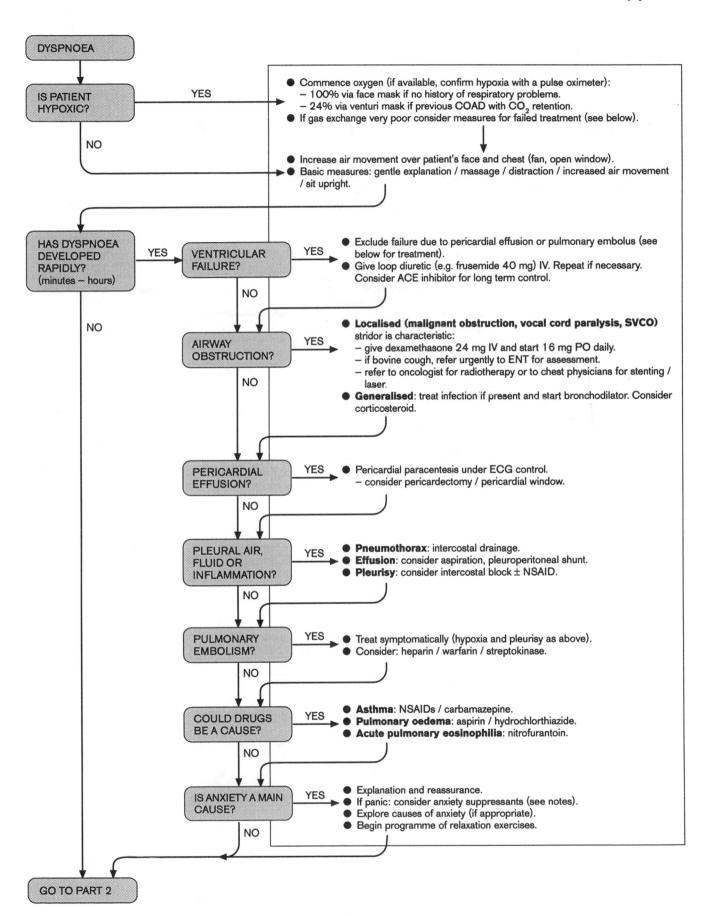

DYSPNOEA

IS PATIENT HYPOXIC? — YES →
- Commence oxygen (if available, confirm hypoxia with a pulse oximeter):
  - 100% via face mask if no history of respiratory problems.
  - 24% via venturi mask if previous COAD with CO_2 retention.
- If gas exchange very poor consider measures for failed treatment (see below).

NO ↓

- Increase air movement over patient's face and chest (fan, open window).
- Basic measures: gentle explanation / massage / distraction / increased air movement / sit upright.

HAS DYSPNOEA DEVELOPED RAPIDLY? (minutes – hours) — YES →

VENTRICULAR FAILURE? — YES →
- Exclude failure due to pericardial effusion or pulmonary embolus (see below for treatment).
- Give loop diuretic (e.g. frusemide 40 mg) IV. Repeat if necessary. Consider ACE inhibitor for long term control.

NO ↓

AIRWAY OBSTRUCTION? — YES →
- **Localised (malignant obstruction, vocal cord paralysis, SVCO)** stridor is characteristic:
  - give dexamethasone 24 mg IV and start 16 mg PO daily.
  - if bovine cough, refer urgently to ENT for assessment.
  - refer to oncologist for radiotherapy or to chest physicians for stenting / laser.
- **Generalised**: treat infection if present and start bronchodilator. Consider corticosteroid.

NO ↓

PERICARDIAL EFFUSION? — YES →
- Pericardial paracentesis under ECG control.
  - consider pericardectomy / pericardial window.

NO ↓

PLEURAL AIR, FLUID OR INFLAMMATION? — YES →
- **Pneumothorax**: intercostal drainage.
- **Effusion**: consider aspiration, pleuroperitoneal shunt.
- **Pleurisy**: consider intercostal block ± NSAID.

NO ↓

PULMONARY EMBOLISM? — YES →
- Treat symptomatically (hypoxia and pleurisy as above).
- Consider: heparin / warfarin / streptokinase.

NO ↓

COULD DRUGS BE A CAUSE? — YES →
- **Asthma**: NSAIDs / carbamazepine.
- **Pulmonary oedema**: aspirin / hydrochlorthiazide.
- **Acute pulmonary eosinophilia**: nitrofurantoin.

NO ↓

IS ANXIETY A MAIN CAUSE? — YES →
- Explanation and reassurance.
- If panic: consider anxiety suppressants (see notes).
- Explore causes of anxiety (if appropriate).
- Begin programme of relaxation exercises.

NO ↓

GO TO PART 2

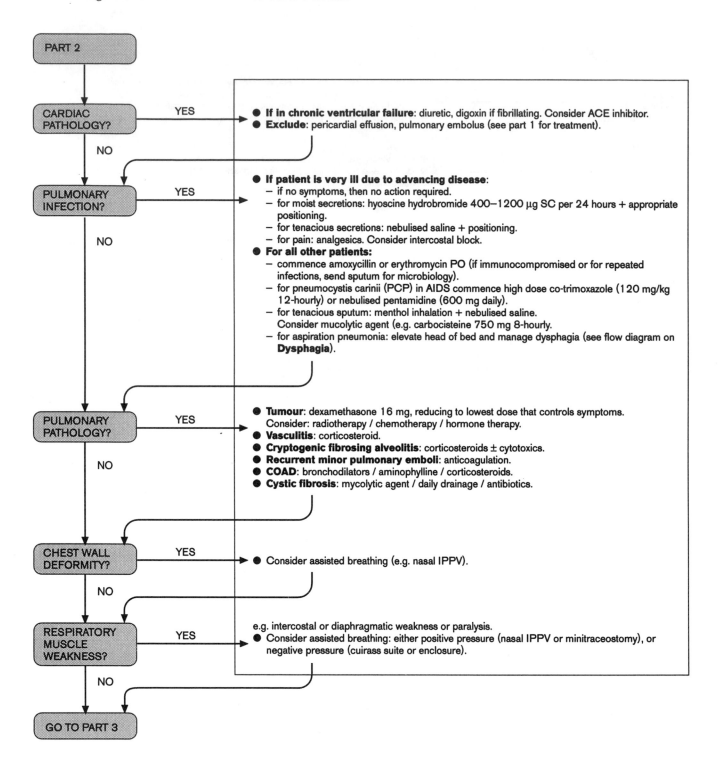

PART 2

CARDIAC PATHOLOGY? — YES →
- **If in chronic ventricular failure**: diuretic, digoxin if fibrillating. Consider ACE inhibitor.
- **Exclude**: pericardial effusion, pulmonary embolus (see part 1 for treatment).

NO ↓

PULMONARY INFECTION? — YES →
- **If patient is very ill due to advancing disease**:
  – if no symptoms, then no action required.
  – for moist secretions: hyoscine hydrobromide 400–1200 µg SC per 24 hours + appropriate positioning.
  – for tenacious secretions: nebulised saline + positioning.
  – for pain: analgesics. Consider intercostal block.
- **For all other patients:**
  – commence amoxycillin or erythromycin PO (if immunocompromised or for repeated infections, send sputum for microbiology).
  – for pneumocystis carinii (PCP) in AIDS commence high dose co-trimoxazole (120 mg/kg 12-hourly) or nebulised pentamidine (600 mg daily).
  – for tenacious sputum: menthol inhalation + nebulised saline. Consider mucolytic agent (e.g. carbocisteine 750 mg 8-hourly.
  – for aspiration pneumonia: elevate head of bed and manage dysphagia (see flow diagram on **Dysphagia**).

NO ↓

PULMONARY PATHOLOGY? — YES →
- **Tumour**: dexamethasone 16 mg, reducing to lowest dose that controls symptoms. Consider: radiotherapy / chemotherapy / hormone therapy.
- **Vasculitis**: corticosteroid.
- **Cryptogenic fibrosing alveolitis**: corticosteroids ± cytotoxics.
- **Recurrent minor pulmonary emboli**: anticoagulation.
- **COAD**: bronchodilators / aminophylline / corticosteroids.
- **Cystic fibrosis**: mycolytic agent / daily drainage / antibiotics.

NO ↓

CHEST WALL DEFORMITY? — YES →
- Consider assisted breathing (e.g. nasal IPPV).

NO ↓

RESPIRATORY MUSCLE WEAKNESS? — YES →
e.g. intercostal or diaphragmatic weakness or paralysis.
- Consider assisted breathing: either positive pressure (nasal IPPV or minitraceostomy), or negative pressure (cuirass suite or enclosure).

NO ↓

GO TO PART 3

Pulmonary embolism: An acute massive pulmonary embolism arising in patients with advanced disease may result in very rapid deterioration for which no specific treatment is appropriate. With a less severe embolism it may be felt reasonable to institute treatment such as immediate heparinisation, but such measures are usually inappropriate in very advanced disease. With recurrent emboli, oral anticoagulation may spare patients the episodes of acute dyspnoea and pain that can accompany such emboli. Recent evidence suggests low dose warfarin is adequate.[3] Pleuritic pain will require analgesics or an intercostal block, and dyspnoea may require pharmacological control (see below).

Pleural effusions can be simply drained using a closed system, consisting of needle, three way tap, collecting bag, syringe and tubing. The use of a small bore suprapubic bladder drainage catheter is an alternative to a needle.[4] If the effusion recurs rapidly and repeated, a pleuroperitoneal shunt should be considered.[5]

Drugs may cause acute breathlessness through an idiosyncratic reaction whose mechanism is uncertain. Depending on the drug, the reaction may be bronchospasm, pulmonary oedema or an eosinophil filled exudate in the alveoli.

Anxiety can be a major contributing factor to some patient's dyspnoea. Counselling and the basic considerations above will be important. Panic may be so severe, however, as to prevent these measures being useful and requiring anxiety suppressant drugs such as lorazepam (0.5–1 mg PO / SL) or the more sedating midazolam (2–10 mg PO / PR / IV). Repeated episodes of panic may respond to relaxation or cognitive therapy.

Slowly developing dyspnoea

When dyspnoea occurs over days or weeks the following may be indicated:

Cardiac pathology: Chronic cardiac failure may be associated with chronic anaemia (see below) or as a late consequence of COAD. Digoxin should only be used in the presence of atrial fibrillation. ACE-inhibitors (e.g. enalopril) are becoming the agents of choice, but have to be monitored on starting as they can cause hypotension, especially in the elderly. Some ACE-inhibitors are also associated with an irritant cough.

Infection producing symptoms are most appropriately treated with oral antibiotics (usually amoxycillin). Alternative treatments should also be considered: hyoscine hydrobromide SC for moist sputum; nebulised saline for tenacious sputum; analgesics or intercostal blocks for pain; and appropriate positioning. Longstanding lung damage, such as bronchiectasis, cystic fibrosis or lung abscess, may require antibiotics active against pseudomonas or anaerobic organisms. Pneumocystis carinii pneumonia (PCP) is common in AIDS and can be treated with antibiotics given orally (e.g. co-trimoxazole, 120 mg/kg 12-hourly) or nebulised (e.g. pentamidine 600 mg daily). Aspiration pneumonia is often overlooked as a cause, as it

may occur silently during sleep in conditions where oesophago- pharyngeal muscle tone is impaired, as in motor neurone disease, or systemic sclerosis (see the flow diagram on *Dysphagia*).

Pulmonary pathology: Dyspnoea due to multiple lung metastases or lymphangitis carcinomatosa may respond to high dose dexamethasone (16 mg daily, reducing to the lowest dose that will control symptoms). Radiotherapy is worth considering for mediastinal lymphadenopathy. Chemotherapy may also be helpful, especially in small cell carcinoma of lung where there can be a 90% response rate. Hormone therapy may also be helpful in breast carcinoma. Pulmonary pathology can also occur as part of a widespread systemic disorder such as systemic sclerosis which may be helped by high dose corticosteroids. Alternatively, conditions may affect the lungs alone as in cryptogenic fibrosing alveolitis which may respond to corticosteroids and/or cytotoxics. Recurrent minor pulmonary emboli can lead to vascular occlusion with ventilation-perfusion mismatching and consequent reduced exercise tolerance. Progression will be slowed or halted with anticoagulation. Airflow obstruction appearing in later life is not usually associated with allergies and is often unrecognised or misdiagnosed as 'bronchitis'. Inhaled bronchodilators and possibly corticosteroids are the mainstay of treatment. Oral xanthine drugs (e.g. aminophylline) are helpful as adjunctive treatments in some patients, but need monitoring because of adverse effects.

Chest wall deformity may be the consequence of old polio, kyphoscoliosis and ankylosing spondylitis. Assisted breathing can be provided by using intermittent positive pressure ventilation (IPPV). By night this improves oxygen desaturation and by day reduces subjective breathlessness. The apparatus can be triggered by the patient's own weak inspiratory effort, or can be set to work automatically at night.

Chronic intercostal or diaphragmatic weakness may result from motor neurone disease and cause distressing difficulty with inspiration. This may be helped effectively by IPPV. Assisted ventilation through a minitracheostomy is less troublesome and more acceptable than traditional tracheostomy or laryngeal intubation, but is rarely used in advanced disease. With severe skeletal deformity, negative pressure by means of cuirass suits or enclosures can relieve the physical burden of breathing.

Cough: A persistent dry cough can exacerbate dyspnoea and is eased by increasing the humidity of the room air. Alternatives are a single spray of 2% lignocaine every 1–2 hours (this is unlikely to cause difficulties with swallowing), or nebulised lignocaine 2%, 5 ml. via a nebuliser over 15–20 minutes, driven with a high flow electric compressor, or from compressed air. Patients should fast for 1 hour after administration to prevent aspiration.

Red cell pathology: It is reasonable to transfuse a dyspnoeic patient if the haemoglobin is less than 9 g/dl. It is not usual practice to transfuse when the prognosis is short (i.e. a day to day deterioration). Transfusion also

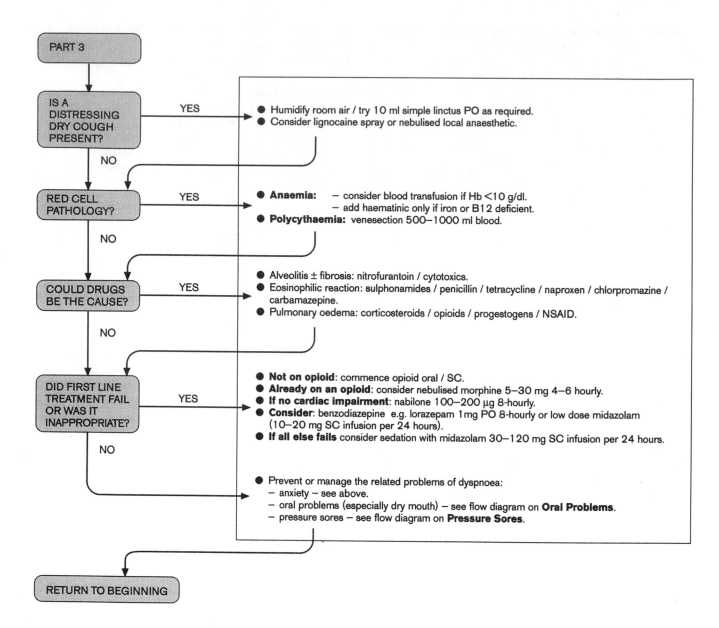

runs the risk of precipitating ventricular failure in elderly patients. Erythropoeitin is helpful in the anaemia of chronic renal failure but is very expensive. Polycythaemia may be secondary to chronic obstructive airways disease and responds well to venesection.

Drugs: The chronic use of some drugs can cause dyspnoea through diffuse lung injury and later fibrosis. Prolonged pulmonary eosinophilia may also occur with some drugs.

Persistent dyspnoea

The treatments above may be unsuccessful or inappropriate. In patients not previously on opioids, morphine or diamorphine can reduce the sensation of dyspnoea in doses of 5–15 mg 4-hourly oral morphine or 10–30 mg per 24 hours diamorphine via SC infusion. Nebulised mor-

phine[6] may also have a role, but must be free of preservatives or additives to be nebulised safely. Diamorphine is widely available in the UK in a form suitable as a nebulised opioid since it is free of preservatives, but its efficacy needs to be evaluated. Nebulised opioids may be more effective in patients with interstitial disease, even in patients already on systemic opioids. In other patients it is worth considering oral nabilone:[7] 100–200 µg 8-hourly. It appears to act by a combination of adrenergic and anticholinergic effects on airways together with a central sedative effect. Nabilone is only available as 1 mg capsules and the lower doses required for dyspnoea will have to specially prepared by the pharmacy. In a few patients, no treatment has been sufficiently effective and they remain severely dyspnoeic at rest with mounting fear and agitation. It may then be appropriate to consider titrated doses of a sedative so that the patient is less aware of his or her surroundings. Ideally this should be done with the patient's permission and that of the patient's family and caring team. Midazolam is the sedative of choice in this situation using 2–10 mg IV or SC, repeated hourly until the patient is settled, followed by 30–180 mg every 24 hours as an SC infusion.

Management of related problems

Dyspnoea can cause secondary problems such as anxiety, oral problems and pressure sores which, if possible should be prevented, but otherwise should be managed appropriately (see the flow diagrams on *Oral Problems* and *Pressure Sores*).

Acknowledgements

We are grateful to Sarah Fitton, nursing sister at St. Oswald's Hospice, for her advice in preparing this flow diagram.

References

1. George PJM, Garrett CPD and Hetzell MR. Role of neodymium YAG laser in the management of tracheal tumours. *Thorax* 1987; **42**: 440–444.

2. Guidelines on the management of asthma. *Thorax* 1993; **48** Suppl.

3. Levine M, Hirsh J, Gent M *et al*. Double-blind randomised trial of very-low-dose warfarin for prevention of thromboembolism in stage IV breast cancer. *Lancet* 1994; **343**: 886–889.

4. Mansi JL and Hanks GW. Drainage of malignant effusions. *Lancet* 1989; ii: 43.

5. Wong PS and Goldstraw P. Pleuroperitoneal shunts. *Br J Hosp Med* 1993; **50**: 16–21.

6. Ahmedzai S. Palliation of respiratory symptoms. In: Doyle D, Hanks G and MacDonald N., eds. *Oxford Textbook of Palliative Medicine*. Oxford: Oxford University Press, 1993;. pp. 349–378.

7. Ahmedzai S, Carter R, Mills RJ and Moram F. Effects of nabilone on pulmonary function. *Proceedings of the Oxford Symposium on Cannabis*. Oxford: IRL Press, 1985;. pp. 371–378.

14 Pressure Sores

Sue Bale
Claud Regnard

The management of a patient with a pressure sore is a complex and difficult management problem. Even with excellent nursing care, pressure sores can develop in the severely debilitated patient. To reduce the likelihood of this happening four issues need to be considered: mobility, pressure relief, nutritional status and local management.

Mobility

Debility, pain, dyspnoea and motor weakness can all result in reduced mobility and increased pressure sore risk. The advice of a physiotherapist is invaluable. See also the flow diagrams on *Dyspnoea*, *Pain* and *Weakness and Fatigue*.

Pressure relief

The patient's environment can be modified using special mattresses,[1] and softer sheets, and by reviewing handling techniques in positioning and turning. Daily assessment of risks (e.g. Waterlow score[2]) and of pressure points will identify those areas in danger (e.g. blanching erythema), so that treatment can be given to avoid more tissue damage.

Nutritional status

If this is appropriate nutritional status should be improved since pressure damage in a poorly nourished patient will fail to heal, or will heal slowly. There are many causes of reduced nutrition in advanced disease: see the flow diagram on *Reduced Nutrition and Hydration*.

Local management

The continuing presence of necrotic tissue creates odour and prevents both healing and the assessment of the degree of damage. Recently, modern dressings have been used to remove necrotic tissue effectively without resorting to surgery, expensive enzymes or chemicals.[3,4] Once debridement is complete, provision of a suitable environment for granulation tissue formation and later re-epithelialisation is required. This environment should:[5]

- maintain a high humidity between the wound and the dressing
- remove excess exudate and toxic components
- provide thermal insulation to the wound surface
- be impermeable to bacteria
- be free from particles and toxic contaminants
- be capable of removal without causing further damage (and hence without pain during dressing changes).

Traditional gauze dressings, antiseptics and hypochlorites do not meet these requirements and should be avoided.[6]

Prognosis

Deciding the prognosis is notoriously difficult. As a rough guide, patients thought to be in the last few weeks of life and deteriorating rapidly (deterioration noticed from day to day) are unlikely to heal anything but the most minor skin damage, and even cleansing may be incomplete. Slower deterioration (week to week) may allow some partial healing of shallow ulcers (< 0.5 cm) if nutrition is adequate, but may allow time only for cleansing with deeper ulcers. Slow deterioration (month to month) may allow time to clean and heal deep ulcers (> 0.5 cm), so long as pressure relief, nutritional status and local management are considered as above.

Care when healing is not possible

There are occasions when the deterioration is rapid, or the poor mobility and nutritional status are irreversible. In such situations pressure sores can develop within days, or existing ulcers can worsen rapidly. A large pressure sore down to bone, for example, is unlikely to heal in a severely debilitated patient, especially if accompanied by osteomyelitis. In this case treatment is best directed towards providing a comfortable dressing and relieving the pain caused by this extensive sore. Odour is managed as in the flow diagram on *Malignant Ulcers*. Any pain is usually from the viable, but damaged, skin at the edge of the ulcer. Good analgesia can be obtained with the topical application of a nonsteroidal antiinflammatory drug (e.g. ibuprofen or benzydamine).[7] For more severe pain, a SC infusion of ketamine, or spinal analgesia can be considered.

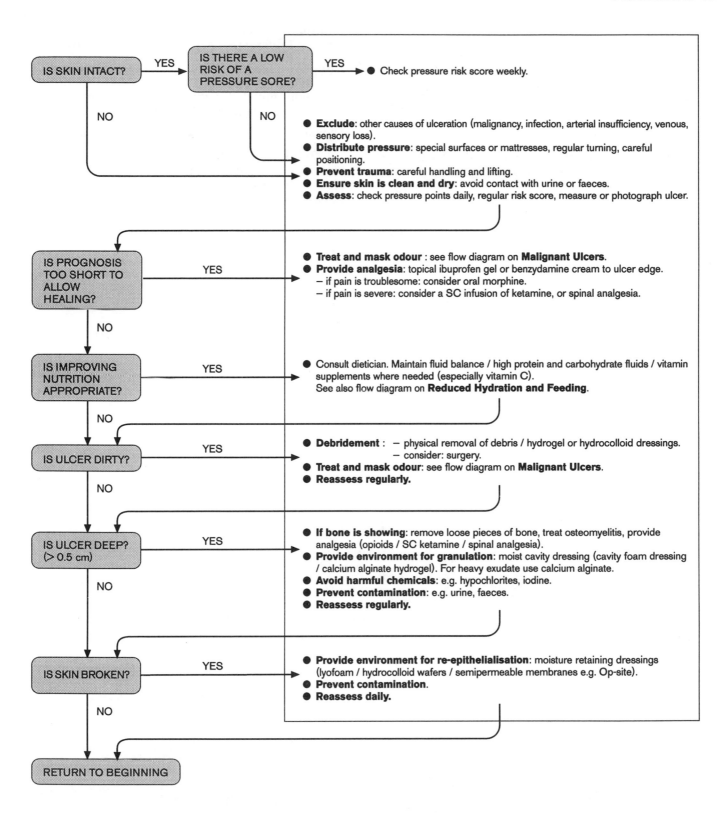

IS SKIN INTACT? — YES → **IS THERE A LOW RISK OF A PRESSURE SORE?** — YES → ● Check pressure risk score weekly.

IS THERE A LOW RISK OF A PRESSURE SORE? — NO →
- **Exclude**: other causes of ulceration (malignancy, infection, arterial insufficiency, venous, sensory loss).
- **Distribute pressure**: special surfaces or mattresses, regular turning, careful positioning.
- **Prevent trauma**: careful handling and lifting.
- **Ensure skin is clean and dry**: avoid contact with urine or faeces.
- **Assess**: check pressure points daily, regular risk score, measure or photograph ulcer.

IS SKIN INTACT? — NO ↓

IS PROGNOSIS TOO SHORT TO ALLOW HEALING? — YES →
- **Treat and mask odour** : see flow diagram on **Malignant Ulcers**.
- **Provide analgesia**: topical ibuprofen gel or benzydamine cream to ulcer edge.
  − if pain is troublesome: consider oral morphine.
  − if pain is severe: consider a SC infusion of ketamine, or spinal analgesia.

IS PROGNOSIS TOO SHORT TO ALLOW HEALING? — NO ↓

IS IMPROVING NUTRITION APPROPRIATE? — YES →
- Consult dietician. Maintain fluid balance / high protein and carbohydrate fluids / vitamin supplements where needed (especially vitamin C).
  See also flow diagram on **Reduced Hydration and Feeding**.

IS IMPROVING NUTRITION APPROPRIATE? — NO ↓

IS ULCER DIRTY? — YES →
- **Debridement** : − physical removal of debris / hydrogel or hydrocolloid dressings.
  − consider: surgery.
- **Treat and mask odour**: see flow diagram on **Malignant Ulcers**.
- **Reassess regularly.**

IS ULCER DIRTY? — NO ↓

IS ULCER DEEP? (> 0.5 cm) — YES →
- **If bone is showing**: remove loose pieces of bone, treat osteomyelitis, provide analgesia (opioids / SC ketamine / spinal analgesia).
- **Provide environment for granulation**: moist cavity dressing (cavity foam dressing / calcium alginate hydrogel). For heavy exudate use calcium alginate.
- **Avoid harmful chemicals**: e.g. hypochlorites, iodine.
- **Prevent contamination**: e.g. urine, faeces.
- **Reassess regularly.**

IS ULCER DEEP? (> 0.5 cm) — NO ↓

IS SKIN BROKEN? — YES →
- **Provide environment for re-epithelialisation**: moisture retaining dressings (lyofoam / hydrocolloid wafers / semipermeable membranes e.g. Op-site).
- **Prevent contamination.**
- **Reassess daily.**

IS SKIN BROKEN? — NO ↓

RETURN TO BEGINNING

References

1. Anonymous. Bedding slants. *Nursing Times* 1994, **90**: 41–51.

2. Waterlow J. The Waterlow card for the prevention and management of pressure sores: towards a pocket policy. *Care – Science and Practice*, 1988; **6**: 8–12.

3. Bale S and Harding KG. Using modern dressings to effect debridement. In: Horne EM, Cowan T. eds. *Staff Nurses Survival Guide*. London: Wolfe Publishing, 1992.

4. Johnson A. Standard protocols for treating open wounds. *Professional Nurse*, 1988; **3**: 498–501.

5. Turner TD. Semiocclusive and occlusive dressings. In: Ryan T (ed) An Environment for Healing: the Role of Occlusion. *Royal Society of Medicine Congress and Symposium Series*, **88**, 1985; pp. 5–14.

6. Thomas S. *Wound Management and Dressings*. London: Pharmaceutical Press, 1990.

7. Jepson BA. Relieving the pain of pressure sores. *Lancet* 1992; **339**: 503–504.

15 Malignant Ulcers

Jackie Saunders
Claud Regnard

A malignant ulcer is defined here as a break in epidermal integrity because of infiltration by malignant cells. This may be due to primary skin malignancy, metastatic deposits or extension of malignancy from deeper structures. For malignant ulcers in the mouth, see the flow diagram on Oral Problems.

Aim of treatment

Simple, basic wound care is recommended for uncomplicated ulcers.[1-4] Each malignant ulcer is unique, requiring individual assessment. Treatment should be realistic and acceptable to the patient and carers. Healing may not be possible when the prognosis is short (day to day, or week to week deterioration), when the primary aim should be to promote comfort and quality of life.

Choice of dressing

The characteristics of an ideal wound dressing to promote healing are well documented.[4] For malignant ulcers we suggest the dressing should:

- absorb excess exudate to prevent maceration of surrounding skin
- not adhere to an ulcer in order to allow pain-free and trauma-free removal
- avoid contamination from external bacterial sources, and be free of nonbiodegradable fibres
- restore/enhance symmetry: by filling cavities with individually moulded wound support products [5] or a fibrous dressing such as Sorbsan; and by reducing bulk with ultra thin dressings over masses. Catering food wrap (Cling Film) can prevent seepage onto clothes
- maintain optimum humidity to prevent painful dry scab formation and aid healing
- protect ulcers from physical trauma
- minimise bleeding
- control or contain malodour
- be cosmetically acceptable to patient and family
- require the fewest possible dressing changes
- maximise patient independence and confidence

Bleeding

Bleeding points can usually be stopped as described. Capillary bleeding can be much reduced with the use of a sucralfate paste applied directly to the ulcer, since it coagulates exposed protein and seals open capillaries. The dressing of choice should ideally remain in place for more than one day; and minimum adherence and totally non-adherent dressings (e.g. Mepitel) can be left in place for up to 7 days with minimum disturbance to the fragile ulcer surface. See the flow diagram on *Bleeding* for more information.

Malodours

These are usually the result of infection with anaerobic bacteria and the odour can be reduced with metronidazole. This can be given as 400–500 mg PO/PR 8-hourly, but nausea can be a problem, in which case topical metronidazole gel is an effective alternative.[6] Masking odours with perfume usually fails since the perfume becomes associated with the unpleasant odour. In contrast, aromatherapy and the vaporisation of essential oils may offer relief.

Psychosocial aspects

Malodour, asymmetry and fear of haemorrhage can cause social isolation, altered body image, sexual difficulties and many other problems.[7] The patient may be too weak to attend a pharmacy personally, or the dressings may not be available on the Drug Tariff. Good communication and planning are essential between hospital, community and hospice, if necessary with one team demonstrating the dressing technique with the other. Consideration should be given to involving the community laundry service if the exudate is excessive and the bed linen is contaminated rapidly. The local authority can also offer a discrete and safe collection service.

MALIGNANT ULCER

IS ULCER BLEEDING? — YES →
- See flow diagram on **Bleeding**.
- Consider radiotherapy or embolisation.

NO ↓

IS AN ALTERED BODY IMAGE PRESENT? — YES →
- **Improve cosmetic appearance**: cosmetic camouflage, disguise cavities with foam or latex dressing, adapted breast prosthesis.
- **Enable to cope with altered image**: acknowledge distress / explore issues (including sexual aspects) / refer for counselling if necessary.

NO ↓

IS ULCER DIRTY? — YES → **WILL PROGNOSIS ALLOW TIME FOR CLEANSING?** — YES →
- **Debride / deslough** gently with polysaccharide, hydrocolloid or hydrogel dressing. Do not use chlorine releasing solutions (e.g. Eusol, Milton).

NO ↓ (from WILL PROGNOSIS ALLOW TIME FOR CLEANSING?)
- **Treat odour**: topical 1% metronidazole gel.
- **Mask odour**: charcoal cloth dressings (e.g. Actisorb, Cliniflex odour control dressing, Lyofoam C) or oxychlorodene (Ostobon) between dressings (not directly on tissues). Cling film (food wrap) can be used to cover dressing to provide extra masking.

NO ↓ (from IS ULCER DIRTY?)

IS DISCHARGE EXCESSIVE? — YES → **IS THIS A SINUS OR FISTULA?** — YES →
- **Reduce volume of discharge**:
  - **if adhesion on flat surface is possible**: paediatric stoma bag.
  - **inflammatory**: topical steroids.
  - **secretory**: topical hyoscine hydrobromide.
  - **urine or faeces**: diversion, e.g. colostomy.

NO ↓ (from IS THIS A SINUS OR FISTULA?)
- **Reduce inflammation**: topical high dose steroids (e.g. Dermovate) once daily for one week. Consider: NSAID or systemic corticosteroids.
- **Absorb discharge**: high absorbency dressings e.g. hydrocellular Allevyn, alginate Kaltostat.
- **Protect surrounding skin**: barrier ointment e.g. zinc ointment.

NO ↓ (from IS DISCHARGE EXCESSIVE?)

IS PAIN PRESENT? — YES →
- **If only at dressing changes**:
  - alternative dressing technique.
  - extra analgesia: additional dose of current analgesic 1 hour before change (not controlled release morphine) / oxygen + nitrous oxide (Entonox) during change / topical local anaesthetic gel.
- **Review systemic analgesia**.
- **Consider**:
  - subcutaneous infusion of ketamine (1–10 mg/kg/24hours).
  - spinal analgesia.

NO ↓

IS ULCER ITCHY? — YES →
- **Remove allergen**: check for allergy to dressing or topical agent.
- **Reduce inflammation**: consider NSAID drug or topical steroids.

NO ↓

RETURN TO BEGINNING

General care

Documentation of size and appearance, using Polaroid prints for example, is valuable in deciding the efficacy of a particular treatment. Compromises may be necessary in some situations: for example, large masses and ulcers producing excessive discharge may require bulky dressings which may be cosmetically unacceptable. It is also important to warn patient and carers of the effects of the treatment chosen. For example, embolisation will initially produce black, necrotic tissue, possibly with some local pain in the first few days; radiotherapy may cause inflammation prior to showing beneficial effects; hydrocolloid dressings (e.g. Granuflex) may appear very dirty after a few days as they take up exudate. It is also important to consult radiotherapy and radiographer colleagues to confirm that the dressing or lotions applied do not contain metals; for example sulphadiazine (Flamazine) contains silver, which will cause radiation to scatter locally with consequent reduced penetration and increased skin sensitivity. Chlorine releasing solutions should no longer be used since they have been shown to stop local blood flow [8] and can damage viable tissue. Large dressings are often most easily handled wearing surgical gloves. Finally, and irrespective of the outcome, the professional should be honest and not show distaste or socially isolate the patient.[9]

Useful addresses

British Red Cross, Beauty Care and Cosmetic Camouflage Service, 9 Grosvenor Crescent, London SW1X 76J, UK.

The Wound Care Society, PO Box 263, Northampton NN3 4UJ, UK.

References

1. Ferguson A. Best performer. *Nursing Times* 1988; **84**: 52–55.
2. Leaper D. Antiseptics and their effect on healing tissue. *Nursing Times*, 1986; **82**: 45–47.
3. Thomas S. Pain and wound management. *Community Outlook* 1989; July 11: 15.
4. Turner TD. Which dressing and why. *Nursing Times*, 1982; **78**: 41–44.
5. Grocott P. The latest on latex. *Nursing Times* 1992; **88**: 61–62.
6. Sparrow G, Minton M, Rubens RD *et al*. Metronidazole in smelly tumours. Lancet, 1980; i: 1185.
7. Clark L. Caring for fungating tumours. *Nursing Times* 1992; **88**: 66–70.
8. Brennan SS, Leaper DJ. The effect of antiseptics on the healing wound: a study using the rabbit ear chamber. *Br J Surg*, 1985; **72**: 780–782.
9. Anonymous. Skin care in palliative care. *Contact: Palliative care nursing group*. RCN 1993; Winter: 6–8.

16 Oedema

Caroline Badger
Claud Regnard

In this flow diagram oedema is defined as an excessive accumulation of tissue fluid, resulting in a measurable swelling. This may be a low protein oedema, a high protein oedema or mixed. Treatment of the disease may improve the oedema, but this flow diagram assumes the progression of the disease is irreversible. Treatment of the oedema therefore includes exercise, skin care and compression or support, and lymph drainage massage.

Many conditions in their late stages may result in oedema. The protein content in these conditions can be either high or low.[1] Low protein oedemas result from conditions causing water accumulation (e.g. cardiac ventricular failure), reduced venous return (e.g. venous thrombosis) or protein loss (e.g. hypoalbuminaemia due to poor nutrition, liver disease or protein losing nephropathy). High protein oedema, or lymphoedema, is usually the result of lymphatic obstruction due to malignancy or the scarring effects of surgery and radiotherapy. Any condition that severely limits limb mobility (e.g. paraplegia due to vertebral metastases, or motor neurone disease) may result in a mixed picture due to venous and lymphatic stasis.

Care of the skin

In venous and mixed oedema the skin is very vulnerable to trauma, particularly if the onset of the oedema has been rapid and acute. If the skin has split or blistered, there is likely to be leakage of tissue fluid from these areas. In contrast, the skin in chronic lymphoedema is usually thickened and dry, and may progress to warty changes and hyperkeratosis, especially in the legs. Hyperkeratosis is less common in arms, but is seen in arm swelling related to breast cancer. Local tumour infiltration gives the skin a characteristic purplish hue. Overnight application of a moisturising cream ensures that any dry skin stays supple. Acute inflammatory episodes, such as cellulitis, are an extremely common complication of lymphoedema and must be avoided as far as possible. Any individual skin breaks must be dressed aseptically, while infected hyperkeratosis requires daily potassium permanganate soaks. If infection is suspected this should be treated promptly with antibiotics. Since streptococcus is the commonest organism, penicillin V is the antibiotic of choice, but if there is no response after 3 days, flucloxacillin should be added. Erythromycin should be used if the patient is allergic to penicillin. Recurrent attacks within one year require long-term treatment with long-term prophylactic antibiotics (e.g. penicillin V 250 mg twice daily), reviewed after three months. Compression hosiery should not be applied to traumatised skin, but bandages can be used until the skin condition improves.

Compression and support[3]

Compression is the deliberate application of pressure derived from the forces inherent in the garment or bandage and is achieved with elastic hosiery or compression bandages. Compression is used when a reduction in oedema is expected or desired, since, as the limb reduces in size, the forces in the garment or bandage pull in to adapt slightly to the reducing limb. In contrast, support is pressure brought about by the tissues of the limb pushing outwards against a garment or bandage. This approach is achieved by wrapping low stretch bandages around the limb (rather than applying them with tension) or by using low pressure elastic hosiery. Support is used when a reduction in oedema is not anticipated or desired, since if the limb were to reduce significantly, the garment or bandage would loosen and fall down.

Bandages are appropriate first line treatment if:
- the skin is fragile, damaged or there is leakage of fluid
- the limb is too large to fit hosiery
- swelling has distorted the shape of the limb
- the limb is too painful to allow the repeated fitting and removal of hosiery
- peripheral arterial circulation is adequate (ankle/brachial arterial pressure ratio of at least 0.75 as measured with a Doppler ultrasound probe)
- cardiac insufficiency is unlikely to be precipitated (if there is a doubt, such patients are best observed as inpatients for the first 48 hours of bandaging)
- at least 8 weeks has elapsed after a venous thrombosis in a leg.

Caution should be taken in the presence of microcirculatory problems (e.g. diabetes), or when sensation is absent.

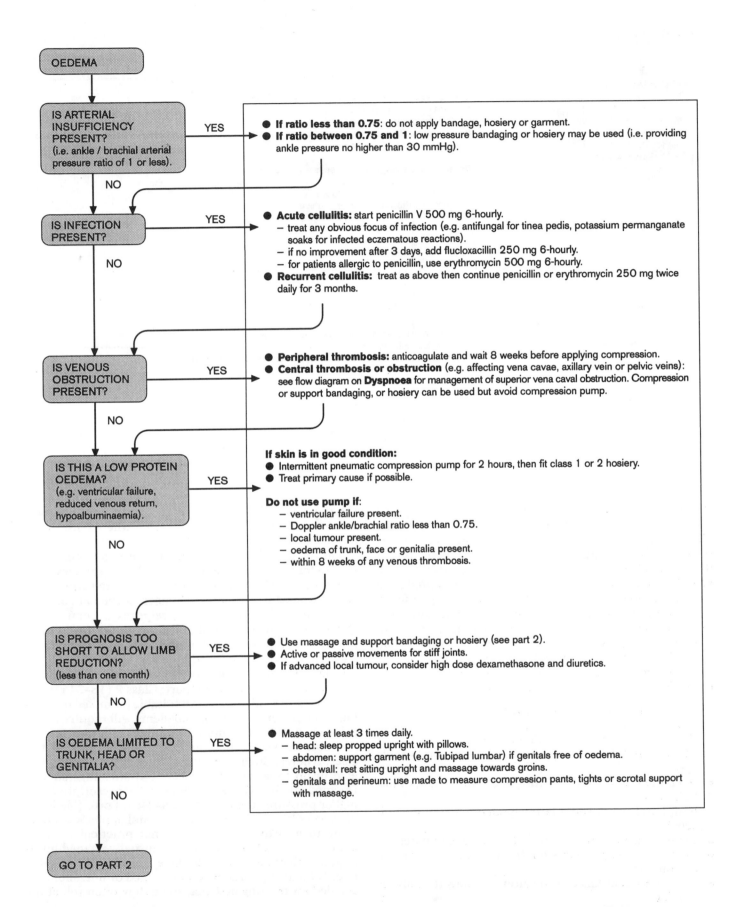

OEDEMA

IS ARTERIAL INSUFFICIENCY PRESENT? (i.e. ankle / brachial arterial pressure ratio of 1 or less). — **YES**

- **If ratio less than 0.75**: do not apply bandage, hosiery or garment.
- **If ratio between 0.75 and 1**: low pressure bandaging or hosiery may be used (i.e. providing ankle pressure no higher than 30 mmHg).

NO

IS INFECTION PRESENT? — **YES**

- **Acute cellulitis**: start penicillin V 500 mg 6-hourly.
  - treat any obvious focus of infection (e.g. antifungal for tinea pedis, potassium permanganate soaks for infected eczematous reactions).
  - if no improvement after 3 days, add flucloxacillin 250 mg 6-hourly.
  - for patients allergic to penicillin, use erythromycin 500 mg 6-hourly.
- **Recurrent cellulitis**: treat as above then continue penicillin or erythromycin 250 mg twice daily for 3 months.

NO

IS VENOUS OBSTRUCTION PRESENT? — **YES**

- **Peripheral thrombosis**: anticoagulate and wait 8 weeks before applying compression.
- **Central thrombosis or obstruction** (e.g. affecting vena cavae, axillary vein or pelvic veins): see flow diagram on **Dyspnoea** for management of superior vena caval obstruction. Compression or support bandaging, or hosiery can be used but avoid compression pump.

NO

IS THIS A LOW PROTEIN OEDEMA? (e.g. ventricular failure, reduced venous return, hypoalbuminaemia). — **YES**

If skin is in good condition:
- Intermittent pneumatic compression pump for 2 hours, then fit class 1 or 2 hosiery.
- Treat primary cause if possible.

Do not use pump if:
  - ventricular failure present.
  - Doppler ankle/brachial ratio less than 0.75.
  - local tumour present.
  - oedema of trunk, face or genitalia present.
  - within 8 weeks of any venous thrombosis.

NO

IS PROGNOSIS TOO SHORT TO ALLOW LIMB REDUCTION? (less than one month) — **YES**

- Use massage and support bandaging or hosiery (see part 2).
- Active or passive movements for stiff joints.
- If advanced local tumour, consider high dose dexamethasone and diuretics.

NO

IS OEDEMA LIMITED TO TRUNK, HEAD OR GENITALIA? — **YES**

- Massage at least 3 times daily.
  - head: sleep propped upright with pillows.
  - abdomen: support garment (e.g. Tubipad lumbar) if genitals free of oedema.
  - chest wall: rest sitting upright and massage towards groins.
  - genitals and perineum: use made to measure compression pants, tights or scrotal support with massage.

NO

GO TO PART 2

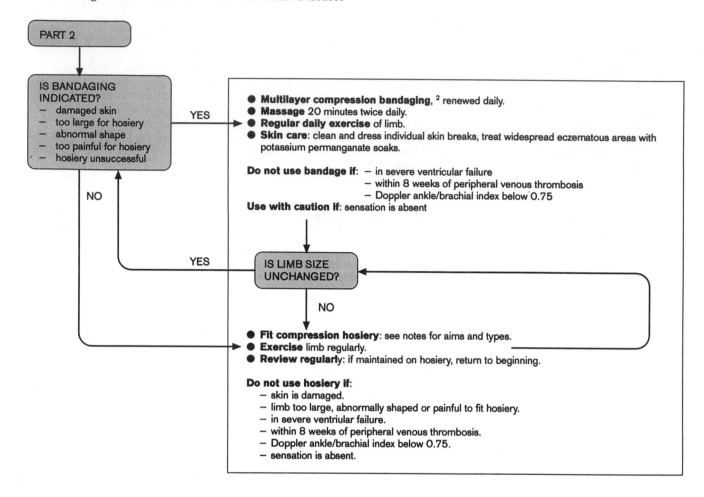

High compression, low stretch bandages such as Comprilan (Beiersdorf) or Rosidal K (Lohmann) are used with the aim of achieving a low resting pressure and a high active pressure. The pressure must be graduated, being higher distally and lower proximally.[4] The medium stretch bandage, Secure Forte (Johnson and Johnson) will produce a smaller difference between resting and active pressures, but has the advantage of being simpler to apply, which is useful if longer term bandaging at home is necessary. Low stretch bandages wrapped around the limb, rather than applied with tension, provide a support bandage (medium or high stretch bandages are not suitable for this purpose). Bandages should be reapplied daily.

Hosiery and garments can be used if:

- the skin is intact
- the limb size and shape will allow fitting
- the limb is sufficiently pain free to allow comfortable fitting
- the patient is capable of fitting and removing it, or has help to do so
- peripheral arterial circulation is adequate (as for bandages)
- cardiac insufficiency is unlikely to be precipitated
- there is enough sensation in the limb to warn of discomfort
- at least 8 weeks has elapsed after a venous thrombosis in a leg.

Caution should be exercised in the presence of microcirculatory problems (e.g. diabetes) or when sensation is absent.

Off the shelf hosiery is available in two compression classes for arms and three classes for legs. Arm sleeves are available short (to the wrist), or with a mitten attached. If hand swelling is present, the longer sleeve is necessary, and hand and finger swelling requires a compression glove (Seton gloves are available in six sizes). Arm sleeves are available through a hospital appliance officer. For legs, the pressure produced by class 1 stockings (10–17 mmHg at the ankle) is only useful for low protein oedemas (e.g. dependency) or for support. Class 2 (18–24 mmHg) and class 3 (25–35 mmHg) are suitable for mixed oedema, but some patients with lymphoedema will require higher pressure hosiery (40 mmHg or more). Classes 1–3 are available in below knee and thigh lengths and in four sizes, whereas higher pressure hosiery is usually available in up to seven sizes. Class 1–3 stockings such as Duomed (Medi UK) are available on GP prescription; but higher pressure stockings such as Medi Forte (Medi UK) have to be obtained through a hospital appliance officer. Made to measure garments are not practical for most patients, but have a place with unusually shaped limbs, although they must be well made and fitted to be effective. Tubular supports, whether shaped or not, should be avoided for treating oedema, since they often roll at one end, producing a tourniquet effect which worsens the oedema.

Massage

This is used for any oedema and is based on the principles of manual lymph drainage.[5] The aim is to move fluid from a congested, oedematous area of the body to one where lymph drainage is normal. The essential principle is to clear the way ahead, so that massage always begins in a healthy quadrant of the trunk, before moving gradually to the swollen side.[5,6] The technique involves stimulating lymphatic drainage by gentle massage of the skin by hand or using an electrical massager. No oil or talc is used before or during massage, so that good skin contact can be maintained. Most patients with obstructive lymphoedema have oedema of the trunk quadrant adjacent to the swollen limb, and concentrating on clearing this congested area helps the limb to drain more efficiently. Even when the limb volume cannot be reduced (e.g. locally advanced breast cancer), this type of massage will help to relieve the feelings of tightness and tension in the oedematous tissues. In these cases the massage will need to be repeated several times a day and may have to be done by a relative or partner. In other cases of lymphoedema, however, massage once or twice daily by the patient is usually sufficient.

Movement and positioning

Patients should be encouraged to use their limbs as normally as possible. Gentle, active exercises whilst wearing some form of compression seem to be particularly beneficial. Elevation should not be considered as a treatment for lymphoedema since it discourages mobility. When the limb is at rest, however, it makes sense to counter the effects of gravity by raising the limb, supported along its full length. A paralysed arm is more comfortable in a supportive sling; the Polysling (Seton) is versatile and widely liked by patients.

Intermittent pneumatic compression pumps

Since these push mainly water back into the capillaries, they can be a useful adjunct to the treatment of low protein oedemas (e.g. hypoalbuminaemia) or mixed oedemas (e.g. immobility) where the problem is largely one of water. Pressures should not exceed 60 mmHg. Multi chamber sequential pumps (e.g. Multicom) may be more effective than single chamber models.

Pumps should *not* be used:

- in patients with ventricular failure (since acute failure can be precipitated)
- with arterial insufficiency (ankle/brachial arterial pressure ratio of less than 0.75)
- in the presence of local tumour
- where there is oedema of the trunk or genitalia
- within 8 weeks of any venous thrombosis.

Measurement

Progress can be most easily monitored with three circumferential measurements at the hand or foot, mid forearm or calf, and at a fixed point in the mid upper arm or thigh. Volume measurements can be made by taking multiple circumferential measurements (a limb measurement pack is available[7]).

Acknowledgements

We are indebted to Peter Mortimer, Consultant Dermatologist, Royal Marsden Hospital, for his advice on the original flow diagram in *Palliative Medicine*.

References

1. Foldi M. Conservative treatment of lymphoedema of the limbs. *Angiology* 1985; **36**: 171–180.

2. Mortimer PS, Badger C and Hall JG. Lymphoedema. In: Doyle D, Hanks G and Macdonald N *Oxford Textbook of Palliative Medicine*. Oxford: Oxford University Press 1993; pp. 407–415.

3. Thomas S. Bandages and bandaging. *Nursing Standard* 1990; 4(supplement): 4–6.

4. Badger C. External compression and support in the management of chronic oedema. In: *The Royal Marsden Hospital Manual of Clinical Nursing Procedures, 3rd edition*. Oxford: Blackwell Scientific Publications; 1992.

5. Földi E, Földi M and Clodius L. The lymphoedema chaos: a lancet. *Annals Plas Surg* 1989; **22**: 505–515.

6. Regnard C, Badger C, Mortimer P. *Lymphoedema: advice on treatment, 2nd edition*. Beaconsfield: Beaconsfield Publishers, 1990.

7. Limb measurement pack. Available from Formword Ltd: 5, Rectory Drive, Gosforth, Newcastle-upon-Tyne NE3 1XU.

17 Weakness and Fatigue

Claud Regnard
Kathryn Mannix

Weakness and fatigue are common complaints in patients with advanced disease and have a wide variety of causes. This flow diagram describes the decisions required to assess the cause, and outlines treatment.

Introduction

The words drowsiness, tiredness, lethargy, fatigue and weakness have different meanings to different patients. Drowsiness usually means an impairment of cognition, such as the reduced alertness caused by sedative drugs. Tiredness is sometimes used in place of drowsiness, or, like the words lethargy, fatigue and weakness, used to describe a general reduction in energy. Weakness is also used by patients to describe a localised motor weakness, although occasionally they may use the words fatigue or tiredness. Carers need to be aware of this wide use of definitions by patients. A typical trap is the complaint of 'tired legs' in a patient who turns out to have a treatable spinal cord compression.

Specific causes and their management

Drugs: reduced alertness is most commonly caused by drugs, especially on starting therapy (e.g. opioids, benzodiazepines, tricyclic antidepressants). Tolerance to this effect may occur, especially with opioids, where tolerance to sedation is seen in 5–7 days. Drugs with a long half life (e.g. diazepam, $t_{\frac{1}{2}}$ of 23–48 hours, more in the elderly), will produce increasing sedation over time. Other drugs may cause general muscular weakness through electrolyte disturbances (see below), or through excessive skeletal muscle relaxation (e.g. baclofen). Drug induced weakness or fatigue is treated by reducing the dose or changing to an alternative drug.

Metabolic disturbances may appear rapidly within minutes or hours (e.g. hypoglycaemia, acute adrenal insufficiency, acute hypercapnia), or more slowly over days or weeks (e.g. hyperglycaemia, hypercalcaemia). Many such disturbances are diagnosed by suspicion alone. Hypercalcaemia is the commonest disturbance, occurring in 10% of all cancer patients (solid epithelial tumours such as breast, bronchus, cervix, and haematological malignancies such as myeloma). It may occur in 25% of patients with bronchial carcinoma, and 20% with breast carcinoma. It can present with one or more of the following symptoms: drowsiness, nausea, vomiting, polyuria, thirst or constipation. Treatment can often reverse symptoms and is by rehydration plus a bisphosphonate (pamidronate or clodronate), usually intravenously. If treatment is inappropriate, nausea can be palliated with haloperidol (see the flow diagram on *Nausea and Vomiting),* constipation with rectal measures (see flow diagram on *Constipation),* and a dry mouth by careful mouth care (see the flow diagram on *Mouth Care*).

Electrolyte disturbances may be caused by drugs (e.g. diuretics, corticosteroids); endocrine abnormalities (hypoadrenalism, correction of hyperglycaemia, inappropriate ADH syndrome), organ failure (hepatic or renal failure); or gastrointestinal disturbances (vomiting, diarrhoea, tumour secretions). Hypokalaemia (e.g. due to corticosteroids, loop diuretics) may present as ileus, generalised weakness or proximal weakness. Hyponatraemia often presents with generalised weakness and lethargy. Treatment will depend on the cause.[1]

Tumour load: Weakness and fatigue in cancer patients may be partly mediated by humoral factors produced by the tumour such as tumour necrosis factor – this is known as a paraneoplastic effect. Some patients enjoy a temporary, but worthwhile, increase in energy and wellbeing on low dose dexamethasone (4 mg daily, reducing to 2 mg after one week). If there is no improvement after 14 days the dexamethasone can be stopped without fear of withdrawal problems.

Infections: Acute, repeated or chronic infections can be very debilitating. Immunocompromised patients such as those with AIDS can be particularly affected, especially as they may have more than one focus or organism involved. Antimicrobial therapy may resolve an infection or may have to be continued longterm to suppress the infection (e.g. persistent candida or mycobacteria). In chronic

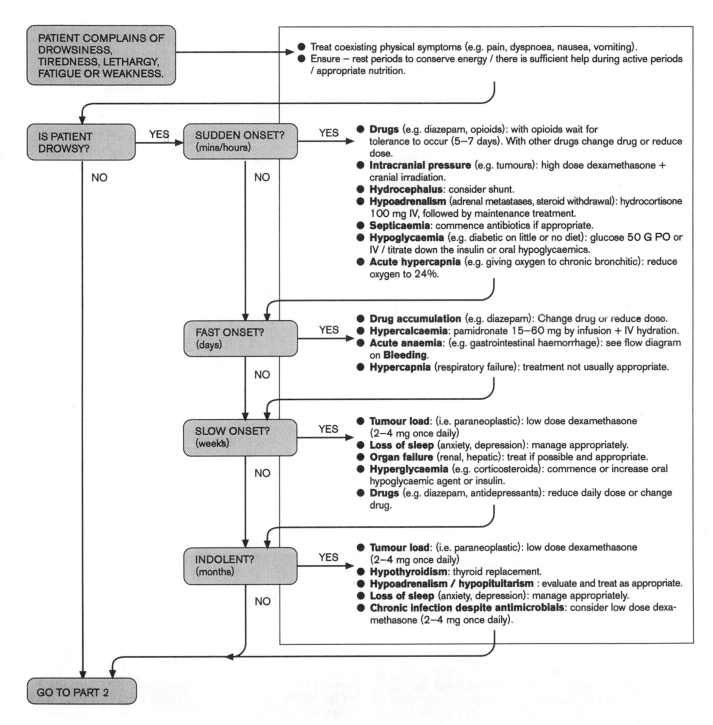

infections, corticosteroids are occasionally used with long term antimicrobials to suppress the undesirable effects of the infection such as pyrexia. If septicaemia is to be treated it is essential that the condition is recognised and treated promptly. Pyrexia may be absent, or hypothermia may be present. There may be a recent history of urinary or chest infections, recent rigors, or the patient may present with lethargy, generalised weakness, drowsiness, confusion, or hypotension. Supportive therapy with parenteral rehydration and antibiotics (if possible chosen from blood or other body fluid cultures) are the

mainstays of treatment. However, severe, acute infection may be a terminal event in patients with advanced disease. In this case, treatment is symptomatic, such as cooling if the patient is pyrexial, analgesics for pain and hyoscine hydrobromide for bronchial secretions.

Anaemia contributes partly to tiredness and fatigue, particularly if the haemoglobin is below 9 g/dl. If there is no symptomatic relief from blood transfusion, this need not be repeated if the haemoglobin drops again. Although the benefit of transfusion may be immediate, stored blood lowers its pH which shifts the oxygen dissociation curve,

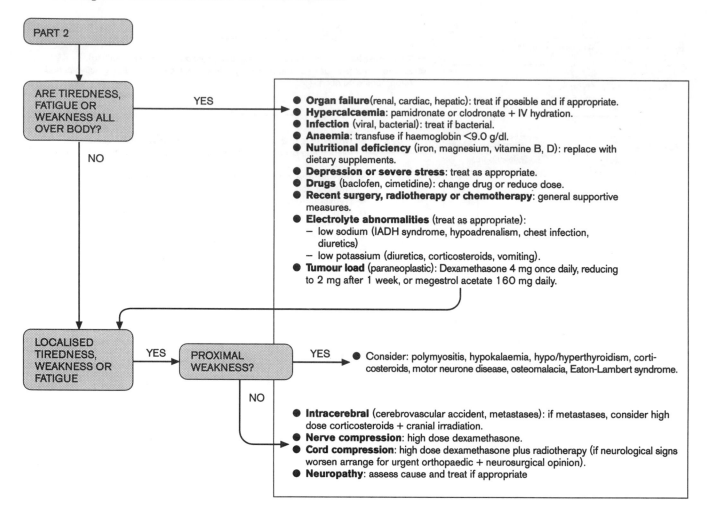

PART 2

ARE TIREDNESS, FATIGUE OR WEAKNESS ALL OVER BODY? — YES →

- **Organ failure** (renal, cardiac, hepatic): treat if possible and if appropriate.
- **Hypercalcaemia**: pamidronate or clodronate + IV hydration.
- **Infection** (viral, bacterial): treat if bacterial.
- **Anaemia**: transfuse if haemoglobin <9.0 g/dl.
- **Nutritional deficiency** (iron, magnesium, vitamine B, D): replace with dietary supplements.
- **Depression or severe stress**: treat as appropriate.
- **Drugs** (baclofen, cimetidine): change drug or reduce dose.
- **Recent surgery, radiotherapy or chemotherapy**: general supportive measures.
- **Electrolyte abnormalities** (treat as appropriate):
  – low sodium (IADH syndrome, hypoadrenalism, chest infection, diuretics)
  – low potassium (diuretics, corticosteroids, vomiting).
- **Tumour load** (paraneoplastic): Dexamethasone 4 mg once daily, reducing to 2 mg after 1 week, or megestrol acetate 160 mg daily.

NO ↓

LOCALISED TIREDNESS, WEAKNESS OR FATIGUE — YES → **PROXIMAL WEAKNESS?** — YES →

- Consider: polymyositis, hypokalaemia, hypo/hyperthyroidism, corticosteroids, motor neurone disease, osteomalacia, Eaton-Lambert syndrome.

NO ↓

- **Intracerebral** (cerebrovascular accident, metastases): if metastases, consider high dose corticosteroids + cranial irradiation.
- **Nerve compression**: high dose dexamethasone.
- **Cord compression**: high dose dexamethasone plus radiotherapy (if neurological signs worsen arrange for urgent orthopaedic + neurosurgical opinion).
- **Neuropathy**: assess cause and treat if appropriate

such that optimum oxygen carriage may not be established for 48–72 hours after transfusion.

Motor weakness affecting skeletal muscle is usually localised to a muscle or muscle groups. Proximal muscle weakness causing difficulty in standing or raising the arms has several possible causes. Examples are polymyositis and Eaton-Lambert syndrome.[2] With localised weakness that also involves distal muscle groups, it is important to exclude spinal cord compression, as any delay may allow cord infarction and irreversible loss of function. Even in a patient deteriorating week by week, treatment may avoid distressing paraplegia and loss of sphincter control, and so maintain the patient's dignity and make care easier in the last stages. An early sign of an increased risk of compression is vertebral pain, usually with local tenderness: pain on coughing or lying flat are particularly important signs. Cord compression may present with limb weakness that may be unilateral. There may be preceding sensory disturbances in the relevant dermatomes, but these may be absent. Conversely, motor signs may be late or absent. Changing neurological function is an important sign, and sphincter disturbance is a late sign. Treatment is with high dose dexamethasone, starting with 24 mg by slow intravenous injection, followed by 16 mg orally per day. The patient should then be referred urgently for radiotherapy. Any deterioration during or soon after this treatment is an indication to consider surgical decompression in appropriate patients. Peripheral nerve compression or damage will produce specific patterns of weakness, depending on the nerve involved, often together with pain. While established damage cannot be reversed, compression may be eased with high dose dexamethasone and/or radiotherapy.

Depression and anxiety: The emotional withdrawal of depression will appear as fatigue to both patient and observers, and may also produce tiredness through loss of sleep. Often mistaken for sadness or paraneoplastic fatigue, depression is underdiagnosed in cancer patients. Anxiety will tire a patient by the constant sympathetic hyperactivity, or through loss of sleep. The use of a Hospital Anxiety and Depression scale is a useful screening measure for both conditions. See the flow diagram on *The Withdrawn Patient* and *The Anxious Person* for details on management.

General care

Some coexisting symptoms, such as pain, nausea, vomiting and dyspnoea, aggravate tiredness and will require treatment. Enabling patients to take frequent rest periods will help them to conserve energy. These rest periods may need to be 'prescribed' by the carer to help family and friends stay away during such periods, and to reduce the frustration some patients feel at being less active. When patients are active it is important to minimise the amount of energy they consume by assessing their mobility needs. When they are inactive, they will need appropriate care to prevent the complications of fatigue (see the flow diagrams on *Constipation* and *Pressure Sores*). Although there is little information available on the nutritional requirements of patients with advanced cancer, it seems reasonable to try to improve their nutritional intake. See the flow diagram on *Reduced Hydration and Feeding*.

References

1. Bower M and Coombes RC. Endocrine and metabolic complications of advanced cancer. In: Doyle D, Hanks G and MacDonald N., eds. *Oxford Textbook of Palliative Medicine*. Oxford: Oxford University Press, 1993; pp. 447–460.

2. Obbens EAMT. Neurological problems in palliative medicine. In: Doyle D, Hanks G and MacDonald N., eds. *Oxford Textbook of Palliative Medicine*. Oxford: Oxford University Press, 1993; pp. 460–472.

3. Zigmond AS and Snaith RP. The hospital anxiety and depression scale. *Acta Psych Scand*, 1983; **67**: 361–70.

18 Confusional States

Averil Stedeford
Claud Regnard

The many potential causes of confusion, and the difficulty of accessing a confused patient, can make this an exceptionally complicated problem to assess, manage and treat. This flow diagram outlines an approach to confusion which emphasises the need to assess fully, treat appropriately and to realise that confusion can be managed even in the face of irreversible causes.

The problems of patients with confusion are exceptionally difficult to elucidate since the carer is often equally confused about what is going on! This is because a number of different psychological symptoms and types of disturbed behaviour are likely to be included under the term, and all of them can be caused by a variety of different physical conditions.

Assessment

Assessment involves the precise identification of the nature of the presenting symptoms and/or behaviours, as well as going through a checklist of likely causes. Often a simple diagnosis cannot be made because the patient may have more than one group of symptoms and also more than one causative condition. By putting the information together, a formulation can be reached which enables further investigation to be done if necessary, and a plan made of treatment of the underlying cause(s) and the management of distressing symptoms. The separation of treatment and management may seem arbitrary, but it serves to emphasise that a great deal can be done to bring relief even when little or nothing specific can be done about the underlying cause. In particular, the right environment, together with adequate explanation to patient, family and staff, are essential elements for successful management.

Memory failure

Recent onset of memory failure is a common component of confusional states. It is likely to be short term or global and results from failure to *take in* information. This type of memory failure is reversible. This is in contrast to

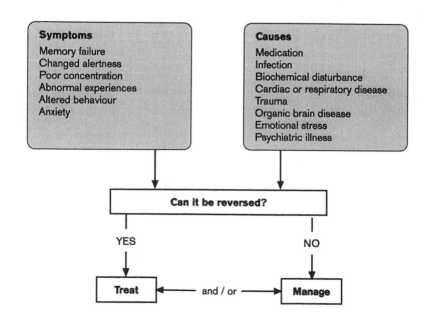

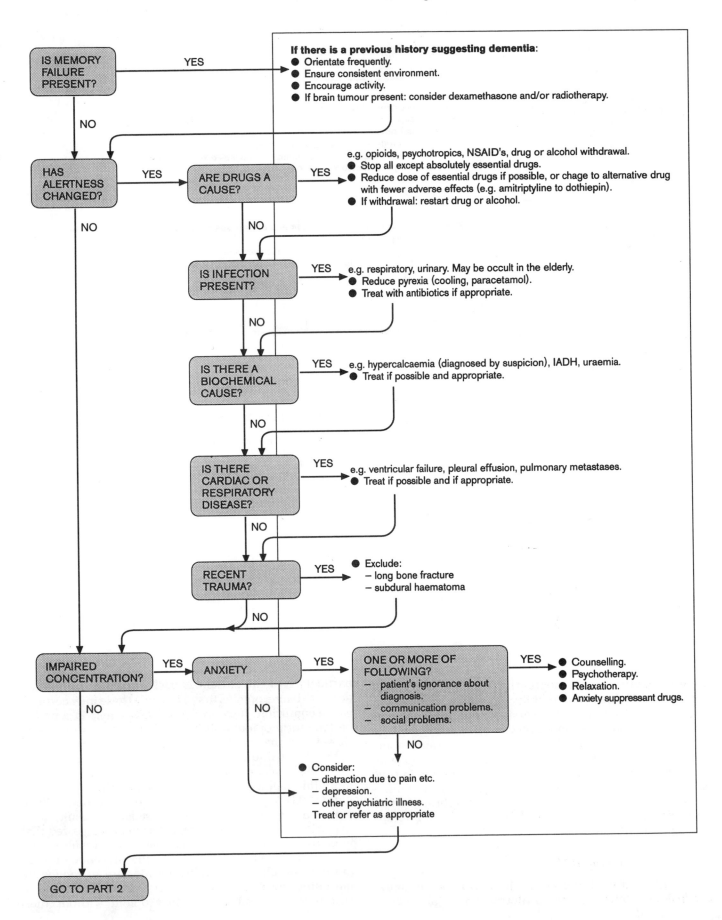

IS MEMORY FAILURE PRESENT? — YES →

If there is a previous history suggesting dementia:
- Orientate frequently.
- Ensure consistent environment.
- Encourage activity.
- If brain tumour present: consider dexamethasone and/or radiotherapy.

NO ↓

HAS ALERTNESS CHANGED? — YES → **ARE DRUGS A CAUSE?** — YES →

e.g. opioids, psychotropics, NSAID's, drug or alcohol withdrawal.
- Stop all except absolutely essential drugs.
- Reduce dose of essential drugs if possible, or chage to alternative drug with fewer adverse effects (e.g. amitriptyline to dothiepin).
- If withdrawal: restart drug or alcohol.

NO ↓ (ARE DRUGS A CAUSE?)

IS INFECTION PRESENT? — YES →

e.g. respiratory, urinary. May be occult in the elderly.
- Reduce pyrexia (cooling, paracetamol).
- Treat with antibiotics if appropriate.

NO ↓

IS THERE A BIOCHEMICAL CAUSE? — YES →

e.g. hypercalcaemia (diagnosed by suspicion), IADH, uraemia.
- Treat if possible and appropriate.

NO ↓

IS THERE CARDIAC OR RESPIRATORY DISEASE? — YES →

e.g. ventricular failure, pleural effusion, pulmonary metastases.
- Treat if possible and if appropriate.

NO ↓

RECENT TRAUMA? — YES →

- Exclude:
  – long bone fracture
  – subdural haematoma

NO ↓

IMPAIRED CONCENTRATION? — YES → **ANXIETY** — YES → **ONE OR MORE OF FOLLOWING?**
- patient's ignorance about diagnosis.
- communication problems.
- social problems.

— YES →
- Counselling.
- Psychotherapy.
- Relaxation.
- Anxiety suppressant drugs.

NO (ANXIETY) →
- Consider:
  – distraction due to pain etc.
  – depression.
  – other psychiatric illness.
  Treat or refer as appropriate

NO (ONE OR MORE OF FOLLOWING?) ↓

NO (HAS ALERTNESS CHANGED?) ↓

NO (IMPAIRED CONCENTRATION?) ↓

GO TO PART 2

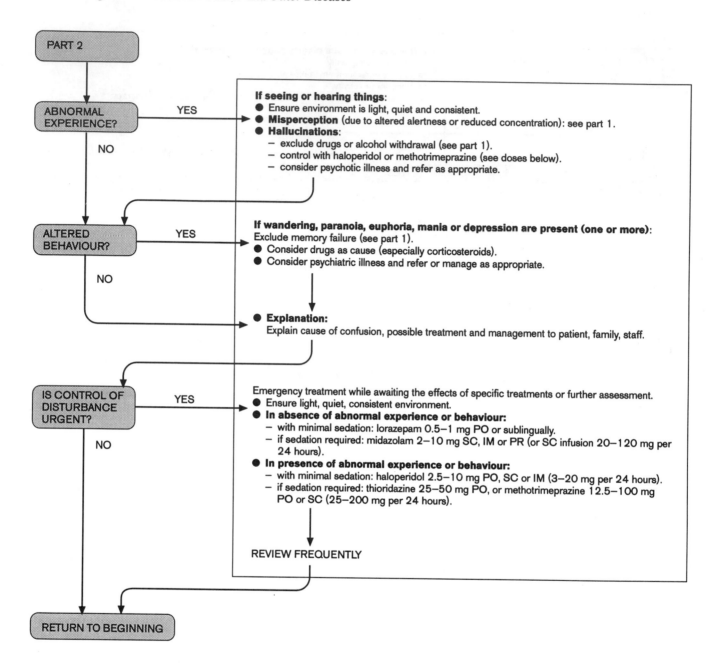

memory failure in the dementias which has a longer history and is due to the inability to *retain* information. Such memory failure is irreversible. The two problems may coexist and early dementia can be unmasked by the stress of serious illness. Patients with cerebral tumours may or may not have memory failure. Patients with memory failure need to be frequently reoriented in time and place, in a light, quiet environment with the minimum of staff changes. The symptoms of cerebral tumours may be helped by corticosteroids[1] or cranial radiotherapy in sensitive tumours.

Alteration in alertness

Although reduced alertness is common in acute confusional states, increased alertness may also occur, particularly if the patient is frightened. There is a tendency to blame opioids first, but while these may certainly cause confusion, they are an unlikely cause in a patient on long term opioids whose renal function is unaltered. However, if the urinary output drops for any reason (e.g. dehydration due to vomiting or reduced intake), then there will be accumulation of the water soluble metabolites morphine-6-glucuronide (M6G) and morphine-3-glucuronide (M3G). M6G is believed to be the active metabolite of morphine and in excess will cause sedation, resulting in a hypoactive confusional state. It has been suggested that, in contrast, excess M3G causes agitation, resulting in a hyperactive confusional state. In the presence of dehydration, therefore, it may be appropriate to reduce the morphine dose. If confusion persists, it is possible to switch to a chemically distinct opioid without these metabolites (e.g. gradually change to methadone starting at a methadone dose of 10% of the morphine dose).

Commonly overlooked drugs are nonsteroidal antiinflammatory drugs, antidepressants, and corticosteroids. Drugs used for urgent control of disturbance may themselves cause confusion, which is why anxiety suppressants and psychotropics should only be used as a last resort (see below). Withdrawal from drugs or alcohol may also cause confusion. Infection is a common cause of confusion in the elderly, in whom the infection may produce few, if any, signs and symptoms. Hypercalcaemia occurs in 5–7% of solid tumours overall but is much more common in certain tumours: it occurs in 20% of breast carcinoma and 25% of bronchial carcinoma. Hypercalcaemia can produce many symptoms (sedation, confusion, nausea, vomiting, constipation, thirst, polyuria); there are no specific signs and the symptoms may occur singly or be masked by other concurrent problems.[2] Previous cardiac disease may be unsuspected and produce ventricular failure. Previous or new respiratory disease may produce hypoxia without warning, and this can be accompanied by marked anxiety.

In patients with unexplained confusion it is therefore important to take a clear history from relatives and friends, including details of any trauma within the past days or weeks. It is necessary to carry out a thorough cardiorespiratory examination, ward test urine for clarity and protein content to exclude infection, and to test blood for electrolytes, together with either ionised calcium or serum calcium and albumin. The speed of resolution of treatable confusion is variable, with most cases taking several days. Some situations may take longer, however, such as confusion due to infection in the elderly, which may take a week or more.

Impaired concentration

This may occur with or without a change in alertness. Anxiety in the presence of ignorance about the diagnosis, communication difficulties with family or care givers, or other social problems, will need one or more of the following: counselling, psychotherapy, anxiety suppressant drugs, or relaxation exercises. Occasionally very severe anxiety can masquerade as depression or so called 'frozen terror'.[3] Reduced concentration may also be due to distraction by physical symptoms such as pain, or due to depression, or another psychiatric illness. The latter may need referral for advice regarding management and treatment. See also the flow diagrams on *The Withdrawn Patient* and *The Anxious Person*.

Abnormal experiences

These may consist of seeing or hearing things, in which case it is important to differentiate between misperceptions and hallucinations.[4] Where a patient has reduced alertness or concentration, misperceptions may occur when an outside stimulus, such as seeing a stranger, is combined with fears or longings, such as the desire to see a daughter, so that the stranger is mistaken for the longed-for daughter. An example is the patient whose alertness is reduced during titration of morphine for pain control. A reduced dose will improve alertness and stop the misperceptions, and a slower titration will allow tolerance to the sedative effect to occur and reduce the likelihood of misperceptions recurring. In contrast, hallucinations have no outside stimulus, being generated internally as a consequence of drugs, alcohol withdrawal or a psychotic illness. An example would be an elderly patient being titrated on morphine who complains of large spiders on the blank wall opposite. Tolerance to this effect does not occur and the morphine dose will have to be reduced and an alternative analgesic or method of pain control will have to be sought. Fortunately this effect of morphine is uncommon.

Altered behaviour

This may consist of aimless wandering, paranoid behaviour (e.g. attempts to 'escape'), paranoid thoughts (e.g. statements about being poisoned), euphoria or mania (e.g. inappropriate gifts or purchases), or depression. Important features of depression in advanced cancer are: persistence of altered mood, loss of self esteem, inappropriate guilt, irritability, diurnal variation of mood and difficulty in accepting help.[5,6] It is important to exclude causes of memory failure (see above), and then to consider other causes such as drugs (e.g. corticosteroids) or psychiatric illness.

Urgent control of disturbance

Even without previous anxiety, confusion is frightening for the patient. It is hardly surprising therefore that some patients become very disturbed at what is happening to them. There is a temptation in such a situation to resort immediately to drugs, but these may themselves worsen the confusion and make access to the patient more difficult. Even very agitated patients will respond to a light, quiet, comforting environment, in which a carer spends time gently exploring what is distressing to the patient. What reassures patients most is a feeling that their carer wants to understand the problem, and knows what to do. This enables the patient to stop worrying without being told to do so!

There are occasions, however, when the disturbance is so severe that access is impossible, or patients are at risk of injuring themselves or others. Medication will then be needed to bring the situation under some control to enable appropriate management to be established. Such patients will need to be reviewed frequently. In the absence of altered behaviour or abnormal experiences midazolam is a useful short acting anxiety suppressant.[7] Lorazepam is an alternative oral preparation with less sedation. Diazepam should be avoided because of its very long half life (7 days in older patients). In the presence of altered behaviour or abnormal experiences an antipsychotic is preferred. Haloperidol causes minimal sedation, while thioridazine or methotrimeprazine can be used if sedation is felt to be necessary.

Haloperidol, thioridazine and methotrimeprazine can be given orally. Midazolam can be given rectally, while midazolam, haloperidol and methotrimeprazine can be given by continuous subcutaneous infusion. Initially the medication should be administered as required with frequent review. In disturbances lasting more than a few hours, however, regular administration may be required, in which case a drug with minimum sedative properties is preferable (lorazepam or haloperidol). A continuous subcutaneous infusion can be used, particularly for midazolam which has a short half life. Haloperidol can also be used this way because sedation is minimal, but continuous infusion with methotrimeprazine, or regular administration of thioridazine should be carefully monitored and reviewed in case the sedation masks a reversible cause. Occasionally a patient is concurrently troubled with nausea and vomiting and this may prompt the selection of an antipsychotic with antiemetic properties (e.g., haloperidol or methotrimeprazine).

Explanation

Explanation is an essential component in managing the confused patient. Explaining the likely cause of confusion to a patient can lessen their anxiety and make it easier to gently explore their worries. This is particularly true when memory failure is present, since many patients fear dementia and 'losing their mind'. It is equally important to provide the family with an explanation since the family too will be frightened by the change in someone they love.

Finally staff will need to understand the reasons for the patient's distress and that the confusion is invariably manageable even if it is irreversible.

References

1. Kirkham SR. The palliation of cerebral tumours with high dose dexamethasone: a review. *Palliative Medicine,* 1988; **2**: 27–33.

2. Heath DA. Hypercalcaemia of malignancy. *Palliative Medicine,* 1989; **3**: 1–11.

3. Brittlebank A and Regnard C. Terror or depression? A case report. *Palliative Medicine,* 1990; **4**: 317–19.

4. Stedeford A. Confusion, in *Facing death: patients, families and professionals, 2nd ed.* Oxford: Sobell publications, 1994; pp. 149–163.

5. Stedeford A. Depression, in *Facing death: patients, families and professionals, 2nd ed.* Oxford: Sobell publications, 1994; pp. 136–139.

6. Stedeford A. Paranoid reactions and other problems, in *Facing death: patients, families and professionals, 2nd ed.* Oxford: Sobell publications, 1994; pp.165–175.

7. McNamara P, Minton M and Twycross RG. Use of midazolam in palliative care. *Palliative Medicine,* 1991; **5**: 249–249.

19 The Anxious Person

Peter Maguire
Ann Faulkner
Claud Regnard

Anxiety can be one aspect of the psychological reaction to advanced disease and may be present at a clinical level. It can hinder or even prevent the diagnosis and management of other problems and when it develops into an anxiety state it can be disabling. This flow diagram describes the key clinical decisions involved in diagnosing and helping a patient or relative troubled with anxiety.

The nature of anxiety

Facing a fear-provoking diagnosis and an uncertain future can cause anxiety as to what will happen in the future and how it will happen. When it becomes obvious that further active treatment is impractical, this anxiety may increase. If an individual looks anxious it is important to identify their concerns, and to differentiate between moderate anxiety (such as the predictable anxiety that occurs as a reaction to the diagnosis) and an anxiety state. Moderate anxiety can be allayed by psychological measures, while a clinical anxiety state will need an active drug regimen. At any level, anxiety reduces the threshold to physical suffering, particularly pain, and hinders the disclosure and resolution of important practical and emotional concerns. It often occurs in association with a depressive illness, and a person with an anxiety state may also have phobic anxiety and/or spontaneous panic disorder. Anxiety that is a natural reaction to an individual's situation can be identified by carefully assessing their problems and concerns. They will report feeling very apprehensive, tense or on edge (see Table 19.1), and will tend to interpret situations and normal sensations in a way that is frightening for them.

Drug induced motor restlessness

For patients, drug induced motor restlessness is an occasional adverse effect of drugs such as prochlorperazine, metoclopramide, haloperidol, methotrimeprazine and chlorpromazine. Because patients are restless and unable to stay still for more than a few seconds they appear tense or on edge, and it is easy to assume they are suffering from anxiety. On questioning, however, it is usually clear that anxiety is not a prominent feature or is even absent, and stopping the drug (or in severe cases giving procyclidine) will soon return the patient to normal.

Table 19.1 Features of anxiety

Apprehensive expectation	Vigilance and scanning
Apprehension	Feeling on edge
Anxiety	Irritable
Worry	Distractible
Fear	Poor concentration
Rumination	Initial insomnia
Dread of misfortune in self or others	Tired on waking
Tendency to perceive situations or objects in a threatening way	Tendency to perceive bodily sensations in a threatening way

Motor tension	Autonomic hyperactivity
Shakiness	Sweating
Jumpiness	Heart pounding
Trembling	Cold clammy hands
Jitteriness	Dry mouth
Tension	Dizziness
Muscle aches	Lightheadedness
Fatiguability	Paraesthesia
Inability to relax	Upset stomach
Restlessness	Hot or cold spells
	Frequent urination
	Diarrhoea
	Lump in throat

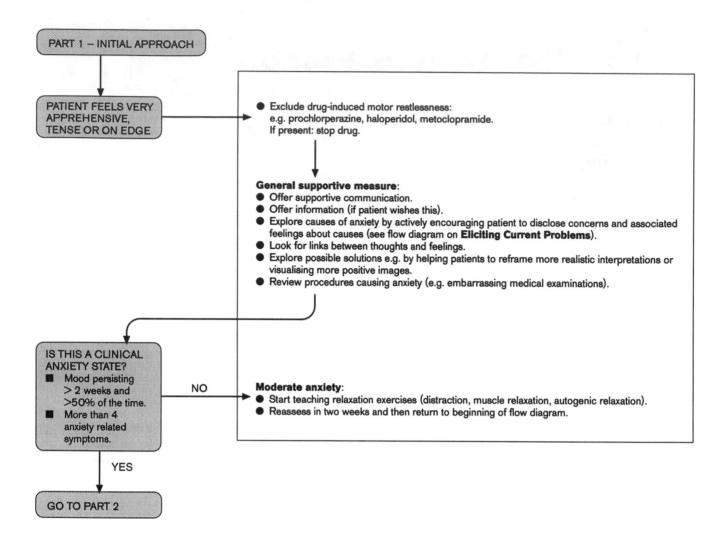

General supportive measures

Allowing a patient to talk about their feelings, or giving them appropriate information and assurance often can reduce the level of anxiety. It is worth trying to deal with any underlying thoughts and feelings that are causing and maintaining the anxiety, to see if these can be resolved. For a more detailed description of eliciting causes, see the flow diagram on *Eliciting the Current Problems*. Possible causes for the patient and relative should be explored and are likely to include fear of the mode of death, physical suffering, uncertainty about the future, loss of role, loss of independence, feeling a burden, spiritual concerns and practical worries like financial difficulties. Where anxiety is related to the patient's uncertainty about the future, it is important to discuss whether they would like markers of progress, such as what symptoms would signal further progression of their illness, since these can provide regular opportunities to discuss progress. It may be possible to help the individual to look for links between thoughts and feelings and to generate more realistic interpretations (e.g. 'I feel out of control with all that machinery.' can be reframed as 'It's good to think all that technology is there to help me.'). Alternatively a person may have a negative image (e.g. 'This chemotherapy feels like they're pouring poison into my veins.'). Through visualisation this can be replaced with a more helpful image (e.g. 'Their drugs are helping to cleanse my body of cancer cells.'). It is also worth reviewing the patient's care, since unthinking approaches can generate anxiety (e.g. asking a shy patient to undress completely prior to an outpatient meeting with the consultant). Thoughtful restructuring of such procedures can greatly ease anxiety. Patients with advanced disease can be kept in a reasonable frame of mind for some considerable time with these strategies.

Moderate anxiety

This will often be helped by taking time to listen, whilst acknowledging the patient's anxiety. Patients and relatives may also be helped by teaching them anxiety management techniques including distraction and relaxation. Muscle relaxation techniques are commonly used, but can worsen the anxiety of those who are excessively vigilant of normal bodily sensations – in these patients autogenic relaxation is safer. This level of anxiety often remits easily, but patients should be monitored to see if they develop a clinical anxiety state.

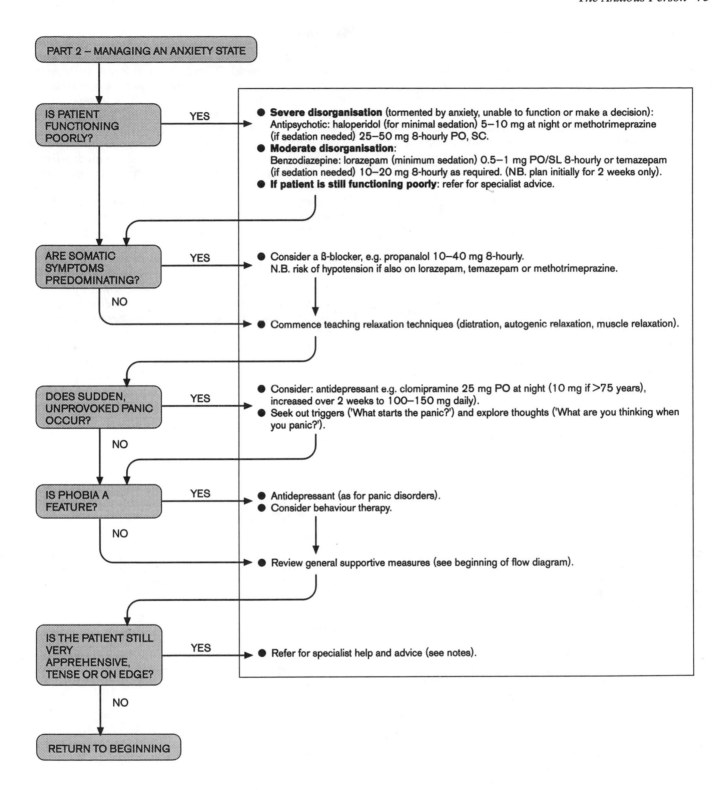

PART 2 – MANAGING AN ANXIETY STATE

IS PATIENT FUNCTIONING POORLY? — **YES**

- **Severe disorganisation** (tormented by anxiety, unable to function or make a decision): Antipsychotic: haloperidol (for minimal sedation) 5–10 mg at night or methotrimeprazine (if sedation needed) 25–50 mg 8-hourly PO, SC.
- **Moderate disorganisation**: Benzodiazepine: lorazepam (minimum sedation) 0.5–1 mg PO/SL 8-hourly or temazepam (if sedation needed) 10–20 mg 8-hourly as required. (NB. plan initially for 2 weeks only).
- **If patient is still functioning poorly**: refer for specialist advice.

ARE SOMATIC SYMPTOMS PREDOMINATING? — **YES** / **NO**

- Consider a ß-blocker, e.g. propanalol 10–40 mg 8-hourly. N.B. risk of hypotension if also on lorazepam, temazepam or methotrimeprazine.

- Commence teaching relaxation techniques (distration, autogenic relaxation, muscle relaxation).

DOES SUDDEN, UNPROVOKED PANIC OCCUR? — **YES** / **NO**

- Consider: antidepressant e.g. clomipramine 25 mg PO at night (10 mg if >75 years), increased over 2 weeks to 100–150 mg daily).
- Seek out triggers ('What starts the panic?') and explore thoughts ('What are you thinking when you panic?').

IS PHOBIA A FEATURE? — **YES** / **NO**

- Antidepressant (as for panic disorders).
- Consider behaviour therapy.

- Review general supportive measures (see beginning of flow diagram).

IS THE PATIENT STILL VERY APPREHENSIVE, TENSE OR ON EDGE? — **YES** / **NO**

- Refer for specialist help and advice (see notes).

RETURN TO BEGINNING

Diagnosing a clinical anxiety state

A clinical anxiety state is present if a patient has felt very apprehensive, tense or on edge for more than two weeks and if this mood disturbance has been present at least 50% of that time. Patients will report that it is significantly different from their normal mood, both qualitatively and quantitatively. Thus, a patient with an anxious personality may normally worry about everything, but will still report a significant and definite increase in the intensity and frequency of anxiety. Importantly, patients with an anxiety state cannot pull themselves out of it or be distracted by others. Thus anxiety of this severity has a dominating and intrusive quality. For a clinical anxiety state to be diagnosed there must also be at least four other symptoms (see Table 19.1). In advanced illness it is important to allow for the possibility that some of the symptoms (such as fatigue and impaired concentration) may be due to the disease.

Is the patient functioning psychologically?

In an anxiety state the anxiety can disorganise a patient psychologically to the extent that it interferes with their everyday ability to function. If the patient is finding it difficult to function and make decisions because of the intensity of the anxiety and is tormented by it, an antipsychotic such as haloperidol or thioridazine should be used immediately. Once the disorganisation has been reduced and the patient is functioning reasonably, it is sensible to offer a benzodiazepine on an 'as needed' basis. A beta blocker such as propanalol should be considered if somatic symptoms predominate. Persistently poor functioning should prompt referral for specialist advice and help.

Panic

The history may reveal that the patient is also suffering from concomitant panic disorder. Here, the patient complains of sudden panic, palpitations, sweating, trembling, depersonalisation and derealisation. These attacks come on suddenly, without warning and without any obvious, external precipitant. They are often intense, lasting 5 to 20 minutes. Their intensity provokes fears of dying and of losing control. When anxiety occurs in the context of a panic disorder, particularly if there is also some depression, it is worth considering using antidepressants such as clomipramine. It is also helpful to seek out what triggers the panic, since this may enable the patient to use coping strategies before the panic develops. Exploring the thoughts going through the patient's mind during the panic attacks may give clues as to the underlying cause.

Phobias

Phobias are irrational fears of specific stimuli which patients try to avoid. There is a tendency to interpret situations or objects as occasions when escape or help is difficult, impossible or embarrassing. Common examples of this include claustrophobia (fear of closed spaces) or excessive fear of objects such as needles, or excessive fear of situations such darkness or chemotherapy. Patients with phobic disorders respond to the same medication as the panic disorders. If phobic patients are well enough they can also be offered behaviour therapy to help with their particular fears. It should be remembered that claustrophobic patients often feel humiliated by their phobia and do not disclose it.

Further support in anxiety states

Once patients begin to function again, teaching patients the relaxation techniques described earlier can be helpful. It is also worthwhile reviewing the general measures described at the beginning of the flow diagram, including activity that encourages patients to disclose their current concerns and associated feelings. By this stage most anxiety states should have responded, but if there has been no response within a week, referral to a specialist is necessary. Help and advice may be needed to

(a) unravel mixed disorders (e.g. alcohol related problems, mixed anxiety and depression)
(b) diagnose unusual presentations of anxiety (e.g. 'frozen terror' [1])
(c) deal with a persisting anxiety state or phobic disorder
(d) provide further counselling of an underlying cause of the anxiety if appropriate and if the prognosis allows.

Specialist advice may be needed from a psychiatrist, psychologist, counsellor or social worker. The patchy distribution of these specialities in some health services means that the final choice may depend on local availability.

Acknowledgement

CR would like to thank Maureen Leyland, Counsellor, St. Oswald's Hospice, for her help and advice with the original flow diagram in *Palliative Medicine*.

References

1. Brittlebank A and Regnard C. Terror or depression? A case report. *Palliative Medicine*, 1990; 4: 317–319.

20 The Withdrawn Patient

Peter Maguire
Ann Faulkner
Claud Regnard

The withdrawn patient challenges effective communication. Some patients are naturally introverted or quiet, but for others the withdrawal represents a change with many possible causes. This flow diagram describes the approach to a withdrawn patient and outlines management.

Possible reasons

When attempting to assess patients with advanced disease it becomes apparent that some are reluctant to talk to you and seem relatively inaccessible. They need to be approached in a non-judgmental way, and consideration should be given to the possible reasons for their apparent lack of cooperation.

Normal behaviour: Patients may be reluctant to talk because they are by nature introverted and loners, and may well appear withdrawn compared to patients who are gregarious. Even if the patient indicates that the withdrawal is normal, it is still worth checking if there are any problems.

Organic cause: The withdrawn behaviour may be a consequence of a confusional state. Such patients will be disorientated in time, place and date and will have difficulty thinking coherently. They experience impaired attention and concentration and may be distractible. Moreover, they may suffer illusions where they misinterpret external stimuli, be hallucinating or even deluded (they may, for example, believe people coming to help them are going to harm them).

In advanced disease likely causes include infection, drugs and metabolic causes such as hypercalcaemia. It is important to check if the patient is orientated to time, place and date by asking the appropriate questions. It is also helpful to check their short term memory by asking them to remember a name and address. Their concentration can be checked by asking them to subtract 7 from 100 and continue to subtract 7 from the resulting numbers. When enquiry confirms an organic confusional state the contribution of psychological factors to withdrawal should still be considered. The clinical decisions and management are described in the flow diagram, *Confusional States*. Drugs may cause withdrawal in a number of ways through sedation (e.g. diazepam), emotional blunting (e.g. chlorpromazine), or tardive dyskinesia

(e.g. metoclopramide, haloperidol, anticholinergics). Withdrawal can also result from cortical damage caused by dementia, or a metabolic cause such as hypothyroidism. Apparent withdrawal can result from aphasia caused by cerebral tumours or a cerebrovascular accident. The cause of the organic diagnosis should be treated if possible, but the remaining management is still appropriate.

Psychological factors

Anger: Patients may feel angry at their predicament. They are likely to be still trying to answer the questions 'why me' and 'why now'? They may be afraid of 'losing control', or their anger may make them feel that talking is a waste of time because it will not cure their disease.

Collusion: The relatives may have insisted that the patient should not be told the truth. Such patients become increasingly isolated from them emotionally and from health professionals. They are frustrated that no one tells them anything, and feel there is no point in trying to establish effective dialogue.

Hidden fears: Patients may be very worried about their predicament, have important unresolved concerns (about their illness and mode of death, or family for example), and yet be reluctant to admit and discuss these because they are so painful. Their withdrawal is then a defence against having to own and discuss their real worries.

Distrust: An important minority of patients with advanced disease will have lost faith in health professionals. They may have been falsely reassured that their prognosis was good or believe that they should have been diagnosed and treated sooner. They have come to distrust health professionals and see no point in talking.

Guilt: Patients can believe that their illness is a just punishment for some past misdemeanour. They may feel that their 'sins' are too wicked to disclose: therefore they do not merit help and are not entitled to burden anyone.

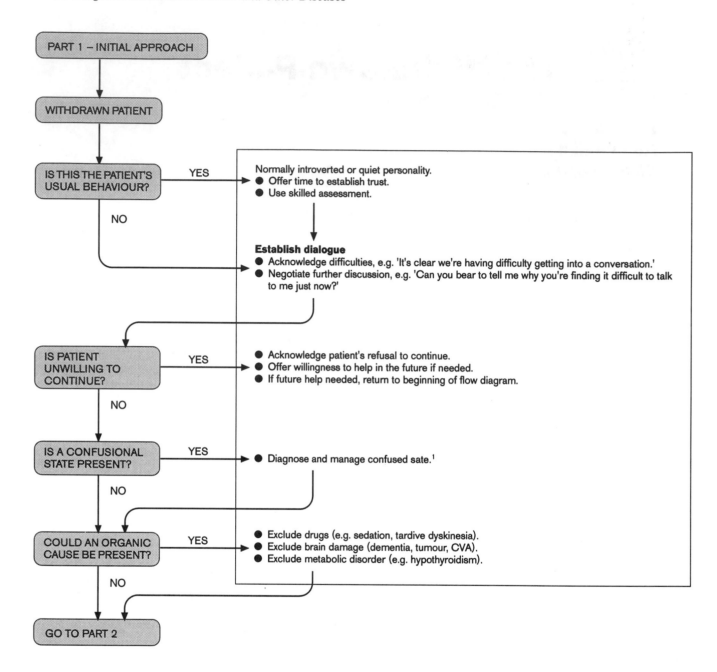

Shame or humiliation: Some patients may be reluctant to talk because they are ashamed of the difficulty they are experiencing in coping with their predicament:

A man in a small four-bedded hospice ward was noticed by the medical and nursing staff to be withdrawn. He had stopped speaking to staff and patients. The staff found it easier to walk past his bed than engage him in conversation. However, subsequent dialogue established that he was full of shame. The shame stemmed from the fact that he had an anal fistula and was repeatedly incontinent of faeces. This caused considerable smell and he was worried this was unacceptable to the other people in the small ward and the staff. He felt that no one understood his problem or was really willing to help. When he admitted this he flooded with tears and

expressed how much embarrassment he felt and how distressing he found it.

Depression: The patient may be suffering from a depressive illness, feel hopeless about the future and believe that nothing can be done to help. Such patients can believe that there is no point in talking as this will not alter the imminence of death. The depression may cause them to feel so apathetic that they do not want to make the effort to talk, concentrate or remember.

Paranoid reactions: Some patients become extremely frightened that others are out to harm them, even when they do not have a confusional state. They are frightened of saying anything in case it is held against them. This may be in the context of a drug induced reaction, depressive illness or other psychiatric illness.

Responding to the withdrawn patient

Confronting the withdrawal: If withdrawn patients are to disclose their problems, this will only happen in an atmosphere of trust. It is tempting for health professionals to believe that they earn trust automatically, but this is not so. Trust has to be earned. You should begin by acknowledging the difficulties you are experiencing in trying to establish a dialogue with the patient by saying, 'As I explained to you I want to talk to you today to find out if you are having any problems that we can help you with. However, it is clear that we are finding it difficult to talk about any problems.' In this way the interviewer acknowledges that this is a problem between them rather than due only to the patient. If the patient is normally very quiet, more time may be needed to establish trust,

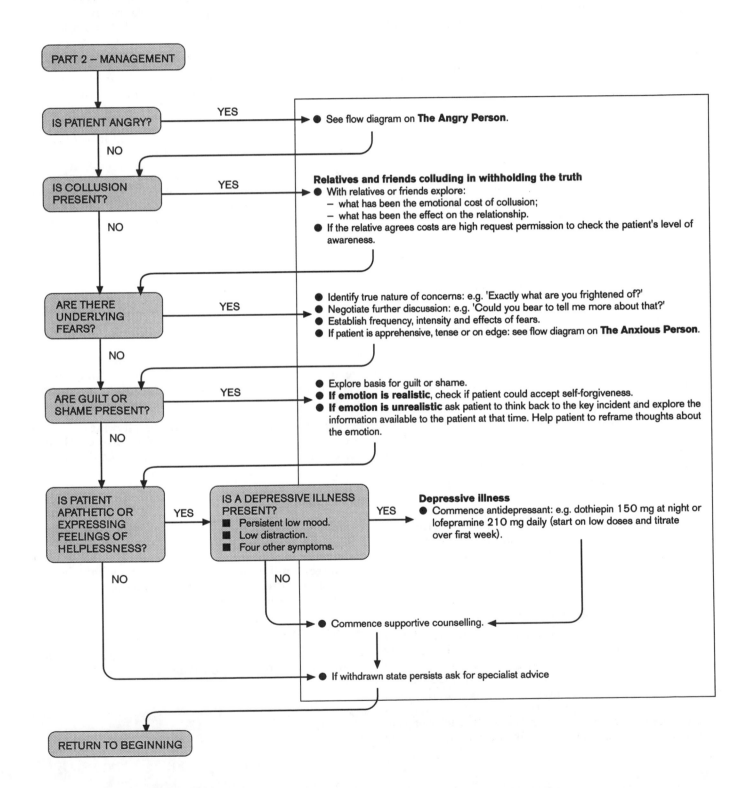

but the problem can be overcome by a skilled approach to assessment and an acceptance of what is 'normal' behaviour for the patient.

To identify the reasons for withdrawal, it is important to negotiate to see if the patient is willing to disclose their difficulties ('Can you bear to tell me why you are finding it difficult to talk to me just now?'). Most patients will respond by giving explicit clues, saying that they see no point in talking, or that no one can change the current situation, or that the health professional could not help them anyway. Patients can then indicate that they have no wish to go further, in which case the dialogue will end there. If the professional now indicates that, although he or she cannot change things, talking might help, then patients may begin to feel that they have nothing to lose by talking to someone who is attempting to understand their concerns. How the rest of the dialogue goes depends on the underlying reasons for the withdrawn behaviour. If it is due to an organic confusional state it should be managed as described in the flow diagram on *Confusional States*.

When the patient indicates that the reason for withdrawal is an underlying fear, the task of the interviewer is to encourage the patient to identify the true nature of the various concerns ('Exactly what are you afraid of?') and negotiate ('Could you bear to tell me more about that?'). It is also important to establish the frequency and intensity of the fears. Thus the interviewer might say 'How often do you worry about this?', 'Just how worried do you get about it?', 'What effect does this have on you?' When it is clear that a patient is very preoccupied with hidden fears, it is important to check whether this has triggered an anxiety state (see the flow diagram on the *Anxious Person*).

Anger: This is more fully explored in the flow diagram on *The Angry Person*.

Collusion: When the withdrawal is the result of relatives and friends deliberately withholding the truth, it is important to talk to them to try to break the collusion. Their reasons for collusion should be explored and the costs of maintaining the pretence established. Collusion is usually entered into in a genuine bid to protect a loved one from suffering. However, it often has significant costs for those colluding, who may find that they are experiencing considerable emotional strain and are also growing apart from the patient because they cannot really share what is happening. If the relative agrees the costs are high, request permission to talk to the patient to check the level of awareness ('I would like to talk to him just to check what he thinks is going on, is that all right?').

Guilt: When a patient indicates that they have withdrawn because they feel guilty, it is important to ask why they are feeling guilty and explore the basis for this guilt in detail. If the guilt is realistic you should check if the patient is prepared to forgive themselves. If the guilt feelings are unrealistic you must insist that they go back to the time of the key incident and look at the information that was then available to them. In this way they should

soon realise that, given the evidence available to them, they had no alternative course of action.

Shame: When shame and humiliation are responsible for withdrawal, it is important to explore, as with anger and guilt, the basis of these feelings and help the patient reappraise their reactions.

Depression: When the withdrawal is due to depressive apathy or feelings of hopelessness, check whether the patient has signs and symptoms of a depressive illness. A depressive illness should be diagnosed if the following three features are present:

1. the patient is suffering from persistent low mood (that is significantly greater quantitatively and qualitatively from the normal mood state) which has continued for at least four weeks for over 50% of the time or all the time for two weeks
2. the patient cannot be distracted out of it by others
3. the presence of four other symptoms.

These symptoms may include diurnal variation of mood (where patients complain they feel particularly worse at some time of the day, usually in the morning), repeated or early morning waking, loss of interest, loss of enjoyment, feelings of hopelessness, feelings of guilt, feeling a burden to others, impaired concentration and lack of energy. When faced with a withdrawn patient who has a depressive illness, it is important to delay counselling until the depressed mood has been alleviated by antidepressant medication. The reason for this is that such patients cannot think positively and may be made worse by counselling at this stage.

Paranoid reactions: It is important to check that these are, or are not, part of a confusional state. If they are not it is important to treat them with appropriate neuroleptic medication or treat the associated depressive illness.

Persistent withdrawal is unusual after following the above, but should trigger a request for specialist psychiatric advice since the cause may be a complicated depression, or a psychosis such as schizophrenia.

Conclusion

Remember that the patient is the only person who really knows the reasons for the withdrawal. Whatever their physical or mental state, most patients are able to identify the reasons for the withdrawal, provided that they are asked about this early on in the encounter and that judgmental statements are avoided.

References

1. Stedeford A. Confusion. In: *Facing death*. London: **2nd edn**. Oxford: Sobell Publications, 1994; pp.149–163.

21 The Angry Person

Ann Faulkner
Peter Maguire
Claud Regnard

Anger from any cause can block effective interaction between the patient or relative and the carer. It has many possible causes which may be rational, irrational (i.e. inappropriate or misdirected), or pathological. This flow diagram suggests strategies for handling anger in patients with advanced disease, their relatives or their partners.

Anger is a common reaction to the knowledge that a disease is advanced and that life expectancy will be shortened. This needs to be acknowledged and the reasons explored with the aim of defusing the anger. If this is not done the anger may build up, explode at a later date and be inappropriately directed. Facing anger can be both draining and upsetting for the health professional, especially if it is unexpected and apparently unjustified. It is important to be non-judgmental when dealing with anger, but also to acknowledge the effects on your own feelings.

Personality

In any assessment a major responsibility is to look for change in an individual. Some individuals have always had an angry approach to life, seeing themselves as one of life's 'victims'. Such people may lack insight into the reality of their behaviour.

Expressions of anger

When anger is actively expressed there is no doubt that the individual is angry. It shows in the use of angry words, tone of voice, facial expression and other non-verbal behaviours. Passive anger presents differently. Passively angry people are very controlled and contained and the initial reaction of the carer may be that they are withdrawn. Careful assessment should reveal the underlying anger.

Whatever the mode of expression of the anger, a key question is whether the anger is proportional to the apparent cause and whether it is directed appropriately.

Situation

It may be that a person is angry for very good reasons which may be unrelated to the illness (e.g. family, financial) or related to the illness (e.g. late diagnosis, delayed referral or lack of information when it was requested).

Unrealised ambitions are common. Few individuals are ready to face death. Many may be angry that they will not have time to realise their ambitions – such as seeing their children grow up, developing their career or reaching certain milestones. This, and spiritual anger, are often accompanied by a sense of guilt, as if the person is taking responsibility for the cancer. This is usually because they are trying to make sense of what appears to be senseless. It is a common belief that cancer equals punishment.

Loss of control is another common cause of anger when patients feel they have been 'taken over' by the illness, by health professionals or their informal carers. This is particularly true when the illness represents a role reversal. For example, the patient may have been the dominant partner throughout married life but now the previously submissive partner has taken on all the major responsibilities. Such anger may be further increased if the patient perceives that their partner can do without them both practically and emotionally.

Feelings of hopelessness may occur when individuals face the reality that they are likely to die. They feel angry at being trapped in a situation from which there seems no escape.

Spiritual causes may be responsible. When facing a fear provoking diagnosis and an uncertain future, many patients begin to question their beliefs. Anger may then be directed at their God with questions such as, 'How can I believe in a God who would do this to me?' Even those who have no religious beliefs may become angry with the unfairness of the situation as they perceive it, e.g. 'I have never harmed anyone – so why should this happen to me?'

Depression may cause the individual to feel angry for similar reasons to the hopeless patient, since it can be difficult to get in touch with any positive feelings. The anger may, however, represent the irritability associated with a depressive illness.

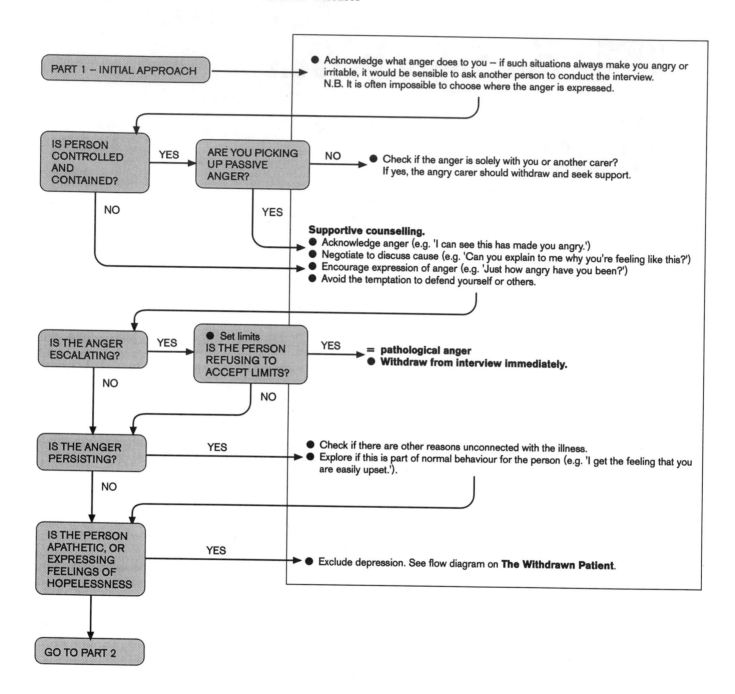

Appropriateness of anger

Rational anger is proportional to the reasons being disclosed and directed appropriately. For example a patient may be angry that a long awaited retirement has now been ruined by the onset of a life-threatening illness. The anger may be self directed, as in the example of a patient with lung cancer saying, 'I always knew I was a fool to smoke, but I didn't believe it could happen to me. I could kick myself now.' To the health professional the level of anger expressed appears in proportion to the cause, and is appropriately directed.

Irrational anger is out of proportion to the reasons being disclosed, or is misdirected, or both. There are many reasons for this irrational anger, but it is often related to the patient or to the feeling that it is not possible or permissible to vent anger where it really belongs e.g. their God, a close friend or relative. The health professional then becomes the target. Self directed guilt and anger can also be inappropriate as in a patient saying, 'I'm so angry at myself. If only I'd been a better person, I'd never have got cancer.'

Rational versus irrational response: At first it may be difficult for the health professional to determine if the expression of anger is rational or irrational. As the reasons for the anger are explored, however, and the verbal expression of anger is encouraged, it should become much clearer. An example of this was a female patient who was angry with her husband for 'not caring enough' about her illness. She gave a rational account of how he had become careless in dress and habits. Only by talking to the husband (smart, clean and concerned) did it become clear that his wife's anger was quite irrational in that she blamed him for being unable to take her cancer away as he was able to take other problems away. By talking to both of them, the true cause of the anger was identified and addressed. With time it becomes easier for the health professional to differentiate between the responses. The health professional soon begins to feel that the amount of anger aimed at them is greater than could be explained by any behaviour of their own. It is not always possible to differentiate between these two types of anger and in cases of doubt it is important to screen for other causes unconnected with the illness, e.g. 'Are there any other reasons why you're feeling angry?'

Pathological anger consists of escalating anger that is out of all proportion to the reasons being disclosed. Usually, the person is visually extremely angry, and may be agitated and pacing about. Anger at this level may increase as soon as the reasons begin to be explored. Since there is a real risk of verbal abuse or physical violence this type of anger must be identified very early in the interview.

Starting by defusing the anger

General: It is important to acknowledge the anger and, when appropriate to acknowledge its legitimacy. This gives individuals permission to express their feelings. Ideally, anger should be acknowledged and explored in private without interruption, but it is not often possible to choose where the anger is expressed. The level of anger will depend very much on the usual behaviour of the individual and their ability to be rational when upset. When the person is rationally angry there is little risk of 'acting out', that is, becoming verbally abusive or physically violent. The key to defusing anger is to acknowledge the anger and to encourage the person to verbalise its cause. If this is done in a non-judgmental way, the anger should defuse as the individual gives it expression. By exploring the cause of the anger, it is possible to make decisions on whether the anger is normal behaviour for that person, and whether it is rational, irrational or pathological. In addition the cause should become clear, such as unrealised ambitions, feelings of loss of control or spiritual issues. Complaints can be a legitimate cause of anger. If the complaint is about the behaviour of a health professional, it is important to avoid the temptation to defend colleagues since this is only likely to spiral the anger upwards, e.g. 'Yes, go on and defend him – you lot all stick together!' It is still possible to show understanding without being defensive, e.g. 'I can see that you are angry that your appointment was delayed – and I guess I would be too.' It is then useful to suggest that the individual tells

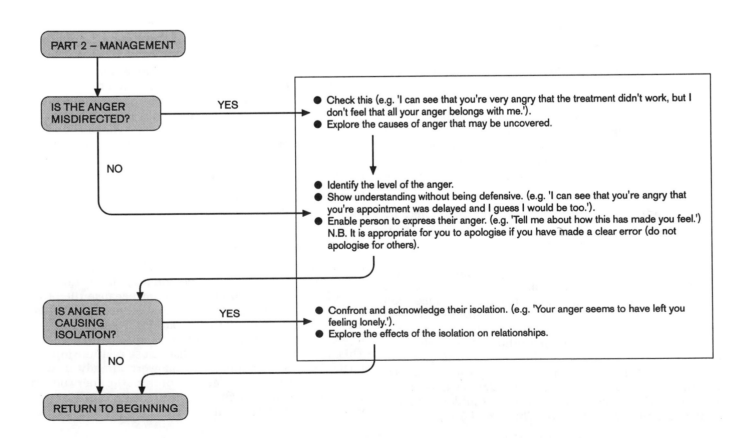

the professional concerned how angry they feel. This can 'clear the air' and allow for proper explanations to be given. However, if the interviewing professional has been involved in a legitimate error, it is important to apologise by saying, for example, 'Yes, I'm afraid we did get it wrong. We did think he would do better than he has done. I'm sorry.'

As the interview proceeds a new phase should begin where the emotions being expressed are now different emotions. These may be feelings of loss about impending death or bereavement, or even guilty feelings. It is then important to explore these feelings and understand their basis.

Persisting anger suggests the cause has not been found and further careful assessment is required.[1] The anger may be irrational, in which case it is crucial to ask whether there could be any other reasons for the anger and to explore these reasons. Alternatively it may become clear that the anger is part of normal behaviour. If this is the case it is still important to acknowledge the anger and to assess the cause and focus of current concerns, since there may be a genuine cause for complaint. It can be worth making an educated guess, 'I get the feeling that you are easily upset.' The reply may be, 'Oh, don't take too much notice of me – I often fly off the handle – but it's soon over.' The patient needs to acknowledge that they are normally angry.

Escalating anger, despite opportunities to disclose the reasons and express the anger, indicates pathological anger and further exploration will be counter-productive. If limits are not set, there is a real risk that the individual will 'act out' by becoming verbally aggressive or physically violent. The health professional should say, 'I can see you're finding it very hard to control your anger. While I don't mind you expressing your anger in words, I can't accept you becoming violent in any way. If you feel you can't give an undertaking about that, then we had better stop the interview right now. On the other hand, if you do feel you can express your anger without losing control, I'd be happy to continue, although I accept you might find that too difficult.' If the person says they cannot control their anger, it is important to insist immediately that the interview is stopped and to leave the room.

Focus of anger: In irrational anger, the focus may be misdirected and health professionals may bear the brunt of much anger that does not belong to them. For example, there is often an angry response from a relative after a patient has been admitted for respite care, and dies within 12 hours. The relative may argue that the patient 'was all right until he came to you'. On the surface such comments seem reasonable, but the health professional should face such misdirected anger sensitively (e.g. 'I can see that you're angry, but I don't think it rests with me.'). It often becomes clear that the anger is the result of feelings of guilt that the relative 'let the patient down' by 'agreeing to respite care'. Similarly, relatives may report anger from the patient that they cannot understand and do not feel that they deserve. This may be because the

patient feels abandoned by the relatives. Health professionals may need to help relatives and others to face the patient. So often, there is the feeling that patients should be treated with kid gloves because they are ill. Just as the health professional can confront misdirected anger, so can the relative (e.g. 'I can see that you are angry darling, but I'm sure I do not deserve your outburst.'). If the patient has insight they may well disclose their real feelings (e.g. 'Sorry love, I shouldn't blame you, but I feel so bitter. I got the feeling you didn't want me any more and just put me in here – I realise I'm being stupid.'). Such sharing can have a major impact on the quality of the relationship during this very difficult period of illness.

Managing the causes of anger

Unrealised ambitions: The nature of the thwarted ambition should be acknowledged and anger legitimised: e.g. 'I can see it must be devastating for you knowing that you will not see your children grow up.' In addition, any feelings of guilt need to be identified and addressed. If the patient can realise that they are not responsible for their predicament, they may begin to forgive themselves and become less angry.

Loss of control: If exploring anger shows that patients feel a loss of control, they can be encouraged to express their feelings and then, when they are calmer, explore ways of regaining some measure of control. It is important that the patient considers solutions themselves rather than have ideas suggested by health professionals which may not be practical or relevant to the individual, e.g. 'I can see your illness has left you with little control. I wonder if you have any ideas for regaining some control over your life?' Reviewing past achievements such as making a life diary, can also be useful.

Spiritual anger: The health professional may feel quite helpless in the face of spiritual anger when the individual's situation *does* seem to be unfair. It is important to take an empathetic approach and acknowledge the difficulty (e.g. 'I can see that it seems unfair, especially when she is so young – it must be very hard for you.'). Such responses can help to defuse the anger. Support from a religious leader may be appropriate.

Depression is managed as described in the flow diagram on *The Withdrawn Patient*.

Managing the effects of anger

Isolation: Anger can cause individuals to distance themselves from others because a person may simply not want to be bothered with anybody else, or because the other people are the focus of the anger. Alternatively others may have less to do with the patient because they are frightened of the anger and uncertain how to respond. This will put strains on previously close relationships, or further impair relationships that were already in difficulty. It is appropriate to gently confront the angry person with their isolation, and to explore the damage this may be doing to the relationships around them. Once this has been established it is useful to consider constructively how they might try to resolve the situation.

Conclusion

Anger should always be acknowledged, legitimised when appropriate, and explored, with the aim of defusing the emotions and moving on to solutions or coping strategies. When the anger persists, the individual should be invited to consider whether there are other reasons that might be causing it other than those so far disclosed. The individual displaying pathological anger should be halted before their anger escalates to violence. No assumptions should be made about the cause, rationality or focus of anger before an assessment is made of each situation. The aftermath of anger may include a variety of emotions that need acknowledgement, but generally the individual needs space to recover before further issues are addressed.

Acknowledgement

CR would like to thank Elspeth Bowden, Macmillan Nurse, for her help and advice in the original flow diagram in *Palliative Medicine*.

References

1. Faulkner A. Handling emotion. In: *Effective Interaction with patients*. Edinburgh: Churchill Livingstone, 1992; pp. 61–68.

22 Breaking Bad News

Ann Faulkner
Peter Maguire
Claud Regnard

Breaking bad news may be necessary at any stage of an illness, and is neither an easy, nor popular task. Properly handled, however, the news can be given in a positive way that the individual can both accept and understand. There will be a range of emotions and concerns following the telling of bad news. These need to be explored and worked through with each individual. This flow diagram describes the steps in this important process.

No one likes breaking bad news. The ancient Greeks always killed the bearers of bad tidings and those feelings that the bad news is linked to the carrier continue today. As a result, many patients and relatives are told bad news by junior doctors. These doctors, who have little experience of dealing with patients, very often tell relatives rather than the patient because they find it easier to break the news at second hand. What they do not consider is the burden that is then put upon the relative to tell the patient. Patients with cancer waiting for the results of tests may themselves be very anxious and worried and not be able to ask about the situation outright. This means that in many cases where there is bad news, both the doctor and the patient or relative are nervous and ill at ease. The key is to break bad news in a way that facilitates acceptance and understanding, while minimising the risk of provoking denial, ambivalence, unrealistic expectations, overwhelming distress or collusion.

Reactions to bad news

There are many reactions to bad news, both at a logical and emotional level.

Acceptance: Many people do accept bad news and adapt to their predicament. They may have had time to prepare for the reality of what they are being told or they may have had some previous experience that has alerted them to the reality of what is happening. Occasionally acceptance may be linked with relief, as the signs and symptoms that have been worrying the person suddenly make sense, perhaps for the first time. It may not be until later that the accepting individual realises the severity of the bad news and shows their reactions by emotions and perhaps tears.

Overwhelming distress: If bad news is broken in the way described below, few patients or relatives will be overwhelmed by their distress. However, this can happen, particularly if the news is broken abruptly without warning. The person will then become extremely upset, weepy or angry. These feelings will be so profound that they are unable to assimilate any subsequent information, or to rescue themselves from their feelings.

Denial: In denial the patient or relative will refuse absolutely to believe the news given. They may go and ask for second opinions from other specialists, and will have a whole host of reasons for refusing to believe that they could possibly be ill. Many such patients will describe themselves as 'fighters':

> 'Nothing like this will ever get me. I know about these things. The doctors have got it all wrong.'

Denial may also show as a complete refusal to talk about the illness and the aftermath. If a health professional tries to talk to such a patient they will simply stop and say to the doctor or nurse:

> 'Look, it's you that's looking after me. I don't want any details, thank you. Just tell me what you're going to do to make me better.'

Ambivalence: The ambivalent person will appear to accept the bad news as it is given. They may give every sign of understanding perfectly what has been said to them. However, the next day the individual may behave as if they simply have not heard the bad news. These individuals go in and out of reality over time, and may spend a considerable amount of time in denial of the facts. If questioned by a health professional about the difference in attitude from one day to the next, this patient will usually have an excuse:

> 'Well, yes, I was pretty low yesterday and the future looked black, but you know, it all looks different today and I'm sure I'm going to get well.'

Unrealistic expectations: The patient or relative with unrealistic expectations will appear to accept their diagnosis from the health professional, but will then describe a number of expectations that simply cannot be met. This

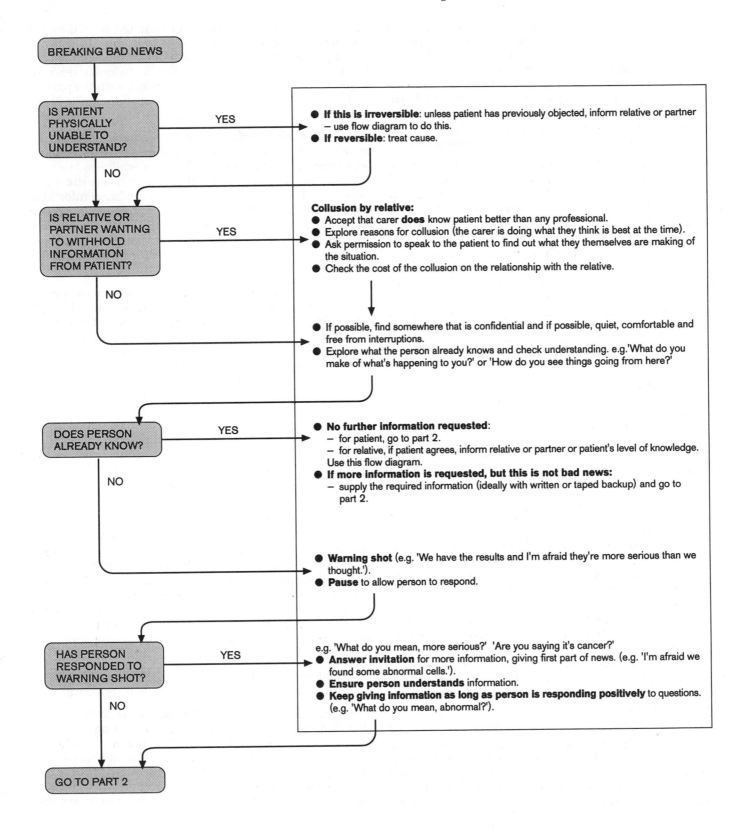

BREAKING BAD NEWS

IS PATIENT PHYSICALLY UNABLE TO UNDERSTAND? — YES →
- **If this is irreversible**: unless patient has previously objected, inform relative or partner – use flow diagram to do this.
- **If reversible**: treat cause.

NO ↓

IS RELATIVE OR PARTNER WANTING TO WITHHOLD INFORMATION FROM PATIENT? — YES →

Collusion by relative:
- Accept that carer **does** know patient better than any professional.
- Explore reasons for collusion (the carer is doing what they think is best at the time).
- Ask permission to speak to the patient to find out what they themselves are making of the situation.
- Check the cost of the collusion on the relationship with the relative.

NO ↓

- If possible, find somewhere that is confidential and if possible, quiet, comfortable and free from interruptions.
- Explore what the person already knows and check understanding. e.g.'What do you make of what's happening to you?' or 'How do you see things going from here?'

DOES PERSON ALREADY KNOW? — YES →
- **No further information requested**:
  – for patient, go to part 2.
  – for relative, if patient agrees, inform relative or partner or patient's level of knowledge. Use this flow diagram.
- **If more information is requested, but this is not bad news:**
  – supply the required information (ideally with written or taped backup) and go to part 2.

NO ↓

- **Warning shot** (e.g. 'We have the results and I'm afraid they're more serious than we thought.').
- **Pause** to allow person to respond.

HAS PERSON RESPONDED TO WARNING SHOT? — YES →
e.g. 'What do you mean, more serious?' 'Are you saying it's cancer?'
- **Answer invitation** for more information, giving first part of news. (e.g. 'I'm afraid we found some abnormal cells.').
- **Ensure person understands** information.
- **Keep giving information as long as person is responding positively** to questions. (e.g. 'What do you mean, abnormal?').

NO ↓

GO TO PART 2

can lead to demands for inappropriate treatment and can cause considerable difficulties. Such unrealistic expectations are possible in both the patient and those who love them. Even when a patient is obviously near to death and no longer able to eat or drink, a relative will often be asking for drips to be put up or for tubes to be put down. These expectations are often linked to denial and any attempt by the patient or relative to accept what is happening results in considerable psychological pain.

Collusion: The breaking of bad news, whether to a patient or a relative, can result in a request from one or the other for collusion. They will argue very cogently that they know the patient or their partner better than anyone in the health care team, and that they know the individual could not take the bad news. There will be considerable pressure to allow the information to be covered up in some way. If the patient asks that others are not told of their diagnosis, this is their legal right, although it can cause problems for the health professionals. If, however, the relative asks that the patient is not told, this causes bigger problems since the patient has a legal right to know their own diagnosis and its prognosis if they wish.

Breaking bad news effectively

Understanding information A patient must be physically capable of understanding information. If this is prevented by confusion due to infection or hypercalcaemia, for example, the cause needs to be treated before attempting to break the bad news. It is possible, however, for the cause to be severe and irreversible (e.g. coma due to end stage disease) or for it to be inappropriate to treat the cause (e.g. obstructive renal failure due to advanced retroperitoneal tumour). Before the deterioration a patient may have made clear his or her objection to information being shared, but this is very unusual. In other cases it is acceptable to inform relatives or partners of the situation, and this is the only situation when such information can be given without the patient's consent. In some irreversible situations such as dementia it may still be possible to give bad news, but this will require careful thought and may need the support and advice of the family or partner. It needs to be remembered that if the relatives or partners are to be told, they will be hearing bad news, therefore this flow diagram also applies to them as well.

Collusion by the relative or partner Even before seeing the patient the health professional may be stopped by a relative or partner (the bottom of the stairs at home is typical). They may ask conspiratorially, 'You won't tell him, will you?' This collusion is usually an act of love: a need for the relative to protect the patient from painful reality. The health professional should always accept that the relative or partner knows the patient much better than anyone in the health care team. The cost of the collusion should then be explored in terms of the emotional strain, and what the impact has been on their relationship. The health professional can then negotiate permission to talk to the patient to find out what they are making of the situation. It is possible in this situation to give a promise that bad news will not be blurted out, but will only be confirmed if the patient is obviously ready to know. By this means it is possible to work with the patient and relative in a useful way, and hopefully bring them together so they can talk through any mutual problems.

Finding an appropriate setting The person should be asked whether they want to move somewhere quieter and who they wish to be present. The place where bad news is broken should be somewhere that cannot be overheard by others, and if possible should also be quiet, comfortable and free of interruptions. It is not acceptable to break bad news in the middle of a busy corridor. The person may wish a friend or relative to be present for support, and may also agree to another professional carer being in attendance.

Finding out what the person knows It is risky to assume how much or how little a person already knows, although up to 80% of patients already realise their disease has recurred or is advanced. They should be asked in a straightforward way, for example, 'What do you make of what's happening to you?', or 'How do you see things going from here?'. Some people will make their knowledge clear and unequivocal, e.g. 'I've got cancer that's spread to the liver – I know time is short.' Others will be more vague, e.g. 'I think it's a cancer', and it will then be necessary to ask what reasons they have for suspecting the cancer. This will usually indicate how aware they are of the situation. When such checking indicates that the person has little awareness it is necessary to move to breaking the bad news.

Breaking the bad news There should be some preparation for breaking bad news. If it comes like a bolt from the sky, the person will find it difficult to come to grips with what they are being told. For this reason, the breaking of bad news should start with a warning shot that provides some indication that the news is not good. For example, opening the front door and seeing a policeman in uniform immediately suggests something bad has happened. The policeman in his uniform is his own warning shot. The health professional will use words as a warning shot:

'We have the results of the tests, Mr. Brown, and I'm afraid they're much more serious than we thought.'

The warning shot will give some indication to the person that they need to come to grips with something that could be unpleasant. It is important that the news, when it follows, is given at the person's pace. The individual who has gone to the doctor with a lump in her breast and perhaps some knowledge of other women who have had cancer, will probably ask for the information straight away:

'You say it's more serious. Are you saying it's cancer?'

Others will not want much information at all, and so what is said should be given at the person's pace. It may be that the person responds to the warning shot by saying:

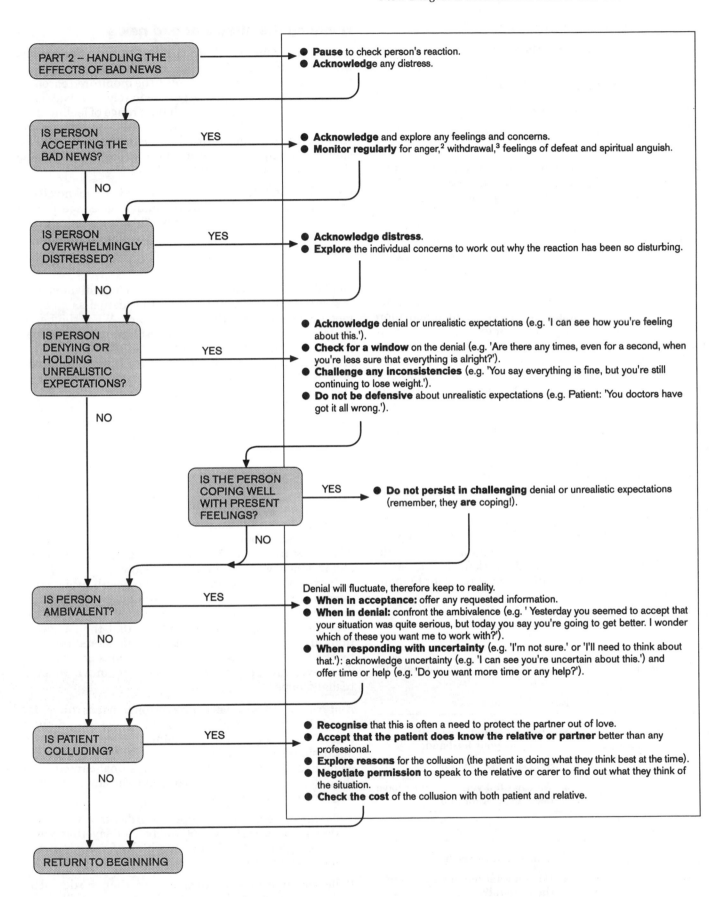

PART 2 – HANDLING THE EFFECTS OF BAD NEWS

- **Pause** to check person's reaction.
- **Acknowledge** any distress.

IS PERSON ACCEPTING THE BAD NEWS?

YES

- **Acknowledge** and explore any feelings and concerns.
- **Monitor regularly** for anger,[2] withdrawal,[3] feelings of defeat and spiritual anguish.

NO

IS PERSON OVERWHELMINGLY DISTRESSED?

YES

- **Acknowledge distress**.
- **Explore** the individual concerns to work out why the reaction has been so disturbing.

NO

IS PERSON DENYING OR HOLDING UNREALISTIC EXPECTATIONS?

YES

- **Acknowledge** denial or unrealistic expectations (e.g. 'I can see how you're feeling about this.').
- **Check for a window** on the denial (e.g. 'Are there any times, even for a second, when you're less sure that everything is alright?').
- **Challenge any inconsistencies** (e.g. 'You say everything is fine, but you're still continuing to lose weight.').
- **Do not be defensive** about unrealistic expectations (e.g. Patient: 'You doctors have got it all wrong.').

NO

IS THE PERSON COPING WELL WITH PRESENT FEELINGS?

YES

- **Do not persist in challenging** denial or unrealistic expectations (remember, they **are** coping!).

NO

IS PERSON AMBIVALENT?

YES

Denial will fluctuate, therefore keep to reality.
- **When in acceptance:** offer any requested information.
- **When in denial:** confront the ambivalence (e.g. ' Yesterday you seemed to accept that your situation was quite serious, but today you say you're going to get better. I wonder which of these you want me to work with?').
- **When responding with uncertainty** (e.g. 'I'm not sure.' or 'I'll need to think about that.'): acknowledge uncertainty (e.g. 'I can see you're uncertain about this.') and offer time or help (e.g. 'Do you want more time or any help?').

NO

IS PATIENT COLLUDING?

YES

- **Recognise** that this is often a need to protect the partner out of love.
- **Accept that the patient does know the relative or partner** better than any professional.
- **Explore reasons** for the collusion (the patient is doing what they think best at the time).
- **Negotiate permission** to speak to the relative or carer to find out what they think of the situation.
- **Check the cost** of the collusion with both patient and relative.

NO

RETURN TO BEGINNING

'What do you mean, more serious?'

The professional carer may then give the first part of the news:

'I'm afraid we found some abnormal cells.'

The person may respond by saying:

'What do you mean, abnormal?', or 'How are you going to make me better?'

After confirming or giving the bad news, it is vital that the health professional pauses to allow the person to respond to what has been said. By giving information at the individual's pace, each person can stop the flow of bad news at any point, effectively saying 'that's enough for today, thank you'. The health professional will need to monitor the situation and continue giving the news as needed. This stage can vary from a few minutes to at least several days.

With people who indicate they wish to hear bad news, the mistake is often made of giving them much more information than they require. If, for example, the patient does have breast cancer, that is the one piece of information she will need. She needs to know what can be done, but at this stage may not want details of all the treatments or options available. These may be raised later according to the temperament of the individual. The health professional needs to give space after breaking bad news for the person to absorb what has happened. It is then important that the health professional picks up the pieces and tries to discover how the person is feeling. It may be that the news is a tremendous shock, in which case the reaction will be one of shock. It may be that they have taken in the most important word to them such as 'cancer', and they will need time for that piece of news to sink in. Table 22.1 shows the steps in breaking bad news.[1] Picking up the pieces may take a considerable amount of time: the individual may need to come back to ask further questions and to ask for other information that is relevant to them.

Table 22.1 Breaking bad news

Strategy	Example
1. Warning shot	• I'm afraid I've some bad news for you.
	Response: Bad news?
2. Bad news (at individual's pace)	• There's been an accident involving your husband.
	Response: How bad is it?
	• We can't tell yet. This must have been a shock for you.
3. Give space	
4. Pick up the pieces	Response: I must see him.
	• Do you want me to take you to the hospital?

Handling the effects of bad news

Acceptance One could argue that if the person accepts the reality, the health professional does not have a problem. In fact, such a person needs to be monitored carefully to see if they need help, if not immediately after bad news, then at a later date. They may have a range of feelings that they work through, including anger, withdrawal, and feelings of defeat and spiritual anguish. The health professional can help by exploring these feelings and helping the individual to work through them.

Overwhelming distress The key here is to acknowledge the distress and then explore the individual concerns that are contributing to the distress. This promotes the expression of the feelings and also allows the health professional to work out why the reaction has been so distressing.

Denial and unrealistic expectations The individual who is firmly in denial may be using that denial as a coping mechanism, and has the right to do so. What the health professional can do is to explore just how the person feels and to pick up the strength of the denial. There are two strategies that can be used. The first is to confront the person with inconsistencies in their history: e.g. 'You say everything's fine, but you're still continuing to lose weight.' The second is to test if there is a 'window' on denial by asking, 'Is there ever a time, even for a second, when you begin to worry that things may not be so straightforward?'. If there is a window, it is necessary to discuss whether they are prepared to look at that reality and talk about it, or whether they prefer to retreat into denial: e.g. 'Are you one of those people who prefers to talk about what's happening to them?' It is necessary to work with the individual at the times when they are feeling a greater sense of reality, but not colluding with them at the times when they are in pure denial. This situation is the same as ambivalence, which is discussed below.

If expectations are unrealistic, the health professional needs to explore with the person what their expectations are, and on what basis they hold them. Very often this dialogue will help the person to see that their expectations are unrealistic. If the health professional responds by challenging the unrealistic expectations and by being defensive, the person is less likely to move to more realistic hopes.

Ambivalence The health professional needs to understand that the ambivalent person is going in and out of denial. It is important to maintain a reality base to discussions so that on days when the patient says they are going to get better, the health professional can confront the difference between the reality and the ambivalence. It may be necessary to say:

'Well, you seemed to accept yesterday that your situation is quite serious, but today you say that you're going to get better. I wonder which of these you wish me to work with?'

If the person responds with an excuse, then the denial has to be accepted at that point. In situations like this, however, the time in denial tends to decrease over time as the patient or relative becomes more convinced of the reality of their situation, and this can be expedited by always staying with the reality that is given in the times of acceptance.

Collusion by the patient Just as with collusion in a relative or partner, when the patient colludes it is usually an act of love driven by the need to protect the partner from painful truths. The approach is the same as in collusion by the relative or partner and aims to bring the couple together so they can talk through any mutual problems.

The individual's perception How individuals view their own circumstances is very important when considering breaking bad news, for no individual comes to a situation in neutral. We all try to make sense of what is going on around us, and we look to past experiences to help us cope with bad news. The person will have looked at signs and symptoms that they have observed and try to put them into some sort of pattern. For example, a lady who has read about breast cancer in a magazine may also have had a family member who had it, so she goes to the doctor expecting bad news. For these reasons, when someone is waiting for news that may be bad, it is always worth asking:

'How does this seem to you?'

Often that individual will reply by saying,

'I'm worried that it's cancer.'

The health professional can then work through with the individual why they think it is cancer and, if necessary, confirm that this is the case.

Communication within the team

Having an additional professional colleague present can be supportive and it will help interprofessional communication if that colleague is from a different discipline. It is essential that a summary of the interview, including the information given, is recorded and included in any correspondence.

References

1. Faulkner A. *Effective interaction with patients*. Edinburgh: Churchill Livingstone; 1992.

23 Handling Difficult Questions

Ann Faulkner
Claud Regnard

Patients with advanced disease and their relatives ask many difficult questions, some of which have painful answers, some of which have answers which contain uncertainty, and some to which there are no answers. They should be able to ask their questions in an environment that allows them to disclose their true worries and have the opportunity to talk them through and to look for options. Health professionals need to develop the relevant skills to help patients and their families to disclose and discuss difficult issues, while handling their own emotions.

When patients are faced with advanced disease and an uncertain prognosis, they often react with a certain level of shock.[1] They may take a varying time to come to grips with reality and indeed may have been so disturbed that any information given to them does not register. A common reaction is for the patient or relative to ask health professionals a series of difficult questions. Some are factual requests, such as whether the treatment will work, whether the patient will make a full recovery, or how long they have left. Other questions may be linked with spiritual beliefs, such as 'why has this happened to me?'

Why are questions difficult?
1. The answer to a question may constitute more bad news and may be seen to take away hope. In this context hope is normally seen in terms of getting better, rather than hope for the best possible future in the time that is left to them.
2. Health professionals often believe that they are expected to have ready answers to patients' questions. This belief often stems from their training and experience. It causes considerable discomfort when a question is asked that does not have a clear answer, such as 'How long have I got?'
3. There may be dissonance between the patient who may want to discuss painful issues, and relatives who may want to collude and maintain unrealistic hope.[1] This situation is seen by many health professions as a conflict of loyalty to the patient and their expressed needs, and the relatives who may have differing needs.
4. It may be difficult to identify what a particular question means. Many participants on workshops have been quite angry that a patient has asked them how long they've got. When they have given as clear an answer as possible they have been surprised to find the patient very upset saying, 'I didn't want you to tell me that'. Understanding the question and its purpose poses a problem for many health professionals.

Hope. In health care, hope as a concept has almost always been seen as hope for a good recovery. This is what health professionals are taught in their training and certainly it is the usual hope of many patients prior to understanding their disease and its prognosis. This rather narrow view overlooks the concept of hope in the short term. If a patient is ready to understand that their life expectancy is much shorter than they thought, then they can be encouraged to look and plan ahead to the time that they have. This will mean looking to achievable goals. Many patients who set short term goals often reach them with a little bit of time to spare, sometimes in spite of a more pessimistic medical opinion. It is very important to understand that the patient is not in neutral over their disease but has ideas and feelings that are often reasonably accurate. Such goals often include meeting major anniversaries or being present at a special event, like the birth of first grandchild.

Uncertainty. Health professionals need to feel secure enough to say 'I don't know', when that is the right and proper answer to a question. If the question is to do with time, or whether the treatment will work, then health professionals need to learn to set markers to give the patient manageable chunks of time. For example, if a patient with lung cancer has few symptoms and is not having treatment, they may be better able to use the time they do have if they have some indication of when or how things will change. They might be told for example, 'You'll know that things are moving on when you get a little more tired'. Other markers can be given that are relevant to each situation. It is very important to recognise how difficult it is for the individual concerned to handle uncertainty because it links with a perceived loss of control which the patient may need to talk through, in order to regain the feeling that they are still able to make decisions and choices.

Dissonance. This may occur when the patient and relative are out of step in what they understand, or want to

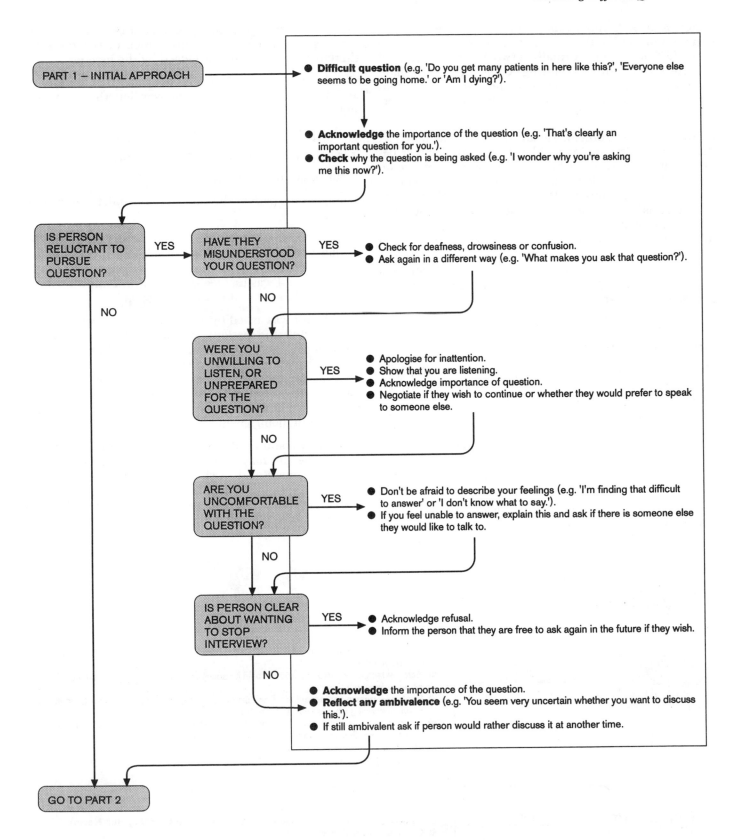

PART 1 – INITIAL APPROACH

● **Difficult question** (e.g. 'Do you get many patients in here like this?', 'Everyone else seems to be going home.' or 'Am I dying?').

● **Acknowledge** the importance of the question (e.g. 'That's clearly an important question for you.').
● **Check** why the question is being asked (e.g. 'I wonder why you're asking me this now?').

IS PERSON RELUCTANT TO PURSUE QUESTION?

YES

HAVE THEY MISUNDERSTOOD YOUR QUESTION?

YES

● Check for deafness, drowsiness or confusion.
● Ask again in a different way (e.g. 'What makes you ask that question?').

NO

NO

WERE YOU UNWILLING TO LISTEN, OR UNPREPARED FOR THE QUESTION?

YES

● Apologise for inattention.
● Show that you are listening.
● Acknowledge importance of question.
● Negotiate if they wish to continue or whether they would prefer to speak to someone else.

NO

ARE YOU UNCOMFORTABLE WITH THE QUESTION?

YES

● Don't be afraid to describe your feelings (e.g. 'I'm finding that difficult to answer' or 'I don't know what to say.').
● If you feel unable to answer, explain this and ask if there is someone else they would like to talk to.

NO

IS PERSON CLEAR ABOUT WANTING TO STOP INTERVIEW?

YES

● Acknowledge refusal.
● Inform the person that they are free to ask again in the future if they wish.

NO

● **Acknowledge** the importance of the question.
● **Reflect any ambivalence** (e.g. 'You seem very uncertain whether you want to discuss this.').
● If still ambivalent ask if person would rather discuss it at another time.

GO TO PART 2

understand. It is important to negotiate with both the patient and the relative to see if there is some common ground.[2] Collusion is normally a two way experience, so the aim of the exercise is getting people together to share their knowledge, their fears and their worries, so that they may be able to move on to making plans for a short term future.

Identifying the problem. Health professionals may feel that there is little point in identifying problems of patients with advanced cancer, since so often there are no ready solutions. Added to this, are all the social implications of talking about difficult areas which may be perceived as 'taboo' such as sexuality, spiritual beliefs and other emotionally loaded areas. A clear distinction needs to be made between professional interaction, and social interaction. The health professional needs to be seen as an individual who will listen to a patient's problems in a non judgmental way, and help them to look at the options and solutions that are open to them, given the uncertainty of their future.

The initial approach

The setting: When a question is asked, the response needs to be in the here and now. If one were to say, 'I'll answer your question, but let's go somewhere quieter', it could well frighten the questioner. It is often necessary to handle difficult questions in circumstances that are far from ideal, such as in the bathroom or the middle of a busy ward, but it is important to remember that the patient or relative is asking because they feel safe enough to ask.

Acknowledge the question: Difficult questions may be difficult for the listener, but for the questioner it has often taken much thought, anxiety and courage, together with trust in the listener. The importance of the question, therefore, must be acknowledged by the listener.

Check the question: This helps to ensure that the listener and questioner are on the same wavelength. If a patient says

'Am I going to get over this?',

it is appropriate to respond by asking

'I wonder why you are asking me that just now?'

This gives the patient the chance to rethink the questions so they may say

'Well, I am asking the question because I get the feeling that you're not going to treat me any more', or they may equally respond by saying, 'Please don't worry about me. I was just feeling a bit low, I know I will get over it. I am planning a holiday soon.'

One doctor was asked by a patient, 'How much longer?', only to find the patient was wanting to know if the outpatient appointment would finish in time for lunch! So by checking why the question is being asked, it is possible for the health professional to discover if the patient wishes to pursue the question and in what way they need information. It also prevents inappropriate information being given.

Does the person want to pursue the question? If there is reluctance, this may simply be due to poor understanding due to deafness or drowsiness. If the person picks up a lack of interest or embarrassment in the listener, they will be reluctant to pursue the matter further. Apologising for the inattention, showing interest and acknowledging the

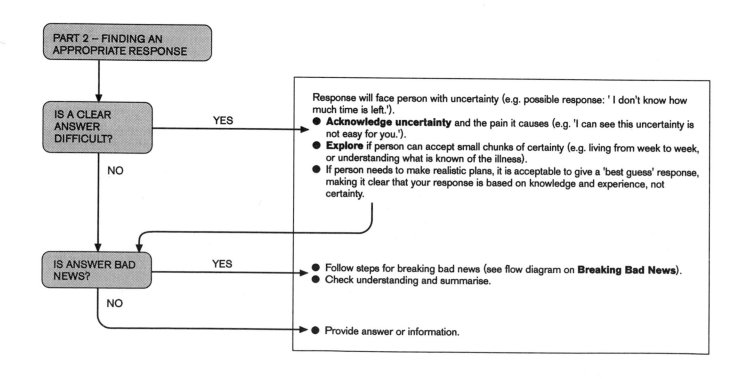

importance of the question again, *may* reassure the questioner sufficiently to continue; otherwise negotiate if they wish to speak to someone else. If the listener feels so uneasy about answering, it is appropriate to admit this and ask if there is someone else the questioner would like to talk to. Of course, having brought the subject into the open, the questioner may immediately decide this is not yet the right time to know. It is then important to acknowledge this and inform them they are welcome to ask again in the future. Alternatively they may be uncertain if they wish to pursue the question- this ambivalence should be reflected and the questioner asked if they would rather discuss it at another time.

Finding an appropriate response

Is there a clear answer? One could argue that every question has an answer but some questions such as 'How long have I got?' are very difficult to answer, since there are so many variables. The straight answer is 'We don't know', but this must be followed by any known probabilities. To say no to a question in a stark way may be very upsetting, so it is useful to ask a subsidiary question such as 'How does it look to you at the moment?' This will often bring a response which shows that the patient is in fact fully aware of how things are and merely wants somebody to confirm it. If the answer to a question constitutes further bad news then one follows the steps for breaking bad news.

Will the response face the questioner with uncertainty? Talking of manageable chunks of time is the aim in dealing with uncertainty, but one has to discover what is a manageable chunk of time for any individual. Some people really can take each day as it comes. Others, however, need much better forecasts so that they can make realistic plans for whatever future is available to them. Some may wish to know whether they have weeks, months or years (specific figures are notoriously inaccurate), while others may wish to know the statstics (e.g. 50% survive 6 months). Most patients accept the impossibility of knowing the exact future, and will respect a carer who is honest enough to say, 'I don't know'.

Communication skills

It will be seen from the above that talking to patients and trying to help them with their difficult questions requires effective communication skills. In particular, it requires that the health professional is able to allow the patient to talk in depth at fairly painful levels. (Table 23.1) Recent research has shown that most health professionals only operate at levels 1 and 2 which allow a patient to give a hint of concern but does not allow them to explore their feelings. This is an area where further work is required.

Table 23.1 Levels of interaction in exploring feelings

Level	Feeling	Example
		Response to 'How are you?'
0	No feeling	'I'm fine.'
1	Hint	'I suppose I'm OK.'
2	Mention of feeling	'I'm worried about my operation.'
3	Feeling expressed	'I'm so worried, I'm having nightmares of me outside my body, disintergrating.'

Acknowledgement

CR would like to thank Richard Gamlin, tutor St. Oswald's Hospice, for his advice.

References

1. Faulkner A. *Effective interaction with patients.* Edinburgh: Churchill Livingstone; 1992.

2. Faulkner A, Maguire P. *Talking to cancer patients and their relatives.* Oxford: Oxford University Press, 1994.

24 Family Problems

Nick Smith
Claud Regnard

The interaction between patient, family and professional team can sometimes be difficult. This flow diagram clarifies the process by which a professional assesses situations and suggests ways in which people can gain understanding about their difficulties. Once everyone has a greater understanding of what is or is not happening, the diagram points to ways in which professionals can use questions to help patient and family create a solution that is workable both for them and for the professionals, and empowers the family.

The effect of crises

Three factors contribute to the family's response to the illness. The *stressor* is the disease itself and creates the current area of concern. The *family's perception* of this stressor is modified by their *existing resources*, such as past experiences, which may strengthen or weaken their ability to cope. Both the event and the family's reaction are further modified by their *current resources*, which may be physical, psychological, social or spiritual. A crisis may bring out the best in people or it may prove the 'last straw'.

Where do you start?

This flow diagram is helpful if you or a member of the family is worried to the point where someone thinks changes need to be made. If a family member has advanced disease the remaining family will not automatically have problems, but how do you know if they are coping? The decisions in this flow diagram will help you since if the answer to all the key questions is 'no', there is no advantage in digging for distress as the family is coping with their situation. A 'yes' answer to any of the questions suggests some further exploration is worthwhile, although listening to the issues may be all that is required. It is helpful to start by drawing a family tree, since it can be used to show relationships in a way that includes the quality of the relationships.

Types of change

When considering the need for change, it is important to distinguish between two types of change we make in our lives. First order change is the most obvious, and occurs when we need to do more of what we are already doing. If a father is not talking enough to his son, for example, he needs to talk more. This can be encouraged by the professional but such change can be very hard for some people, in which case it is necessary to acknowledge the difficulty and offer more specialist help. A second order change is more fundamental. If a relative is threatening violence to another family member, any level of violence would be unacceptable. Changing this behaviour is unlikely to occur except out of desperation or through an acknowledgement that this behaviour has been unhelpful and harmful.

First order change

First order change demands that the family make small adjustments in the way they cope, plan more effectively, try to be less protective, communicate more clearly over specific issues, and get more support and help. A gentle approach is the key.

Is the family coping? Clearly if the family is coping there is usually no need to explore further. Occasionally, however, there is some ambivalence in the answer, and it is worth looking at the strengths that may help them cope. It is rare for members of a family to think the same way about a major issue. It is therefore important to check how each person sees the problem and its possible solution. If the family is seen together, people can be encouraged to exchange views and observed to see if they have the flexibility to problem solve together. If only one family member is present they can be asked what other family members would think if they were there to talk for themselves.

If it is only the professional that is worried, it is legitimate to ask 'what if ' questions:

Professional: 'Have you thought what you would all do if Jean doesn't manage to walk before she goes home?'

Family: 'Well, we just know she's going to walk.'

Professional: 'That would be wonderful, but what if she doesn't?'

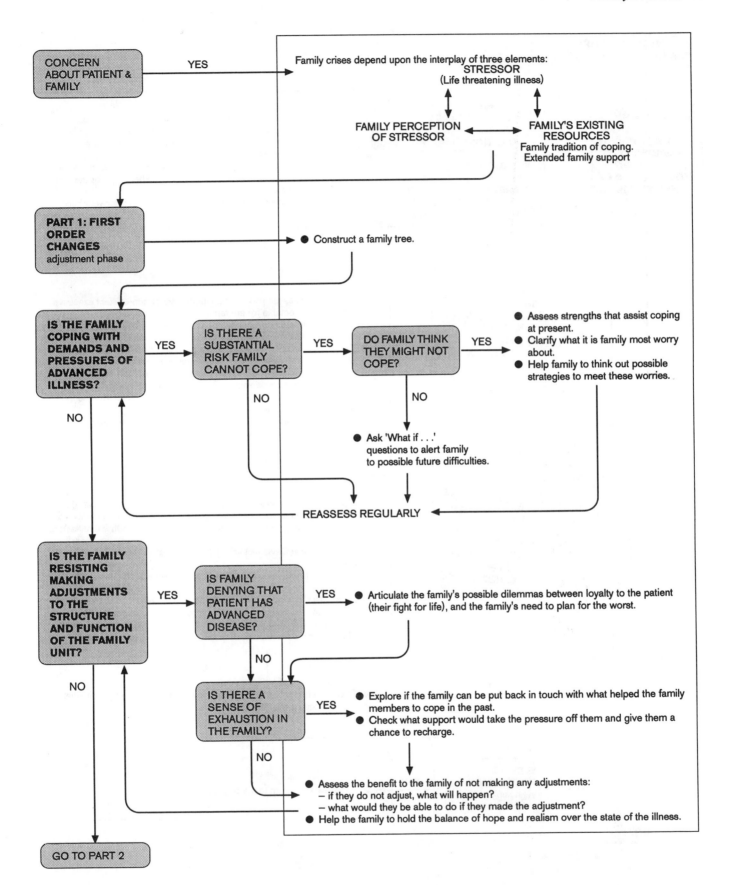

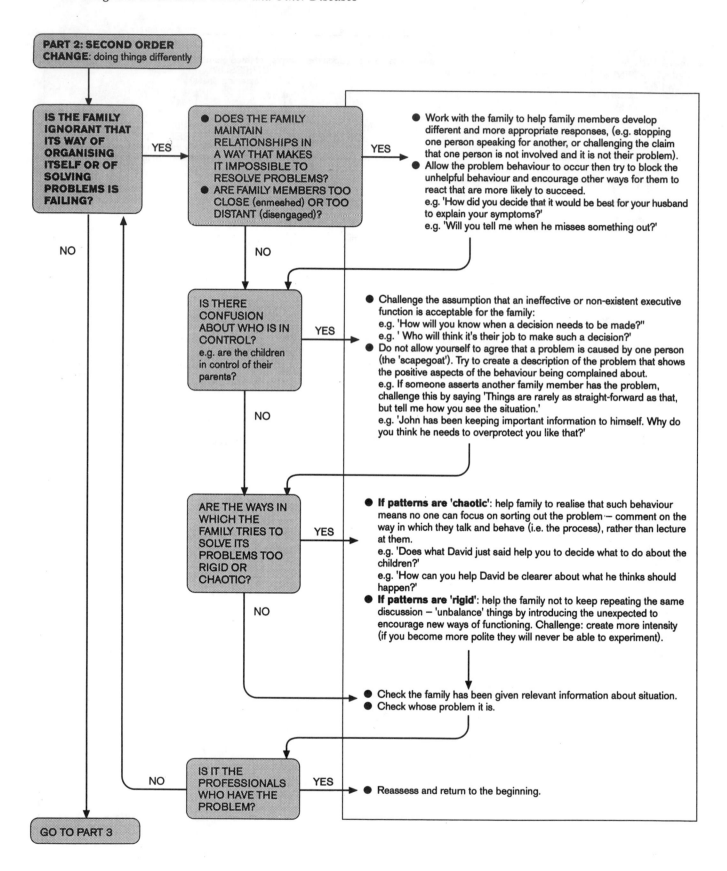

PART 2: SECOND ORDER CHANGE: doing things differently

IS THE FAMILY IGNORANT THAT ITS WAY OF ORGANISING ITSELF OR OF SOLVING PROBLEMS IS FAILING?

YES →

NO

● **DOES THE FAMILY MAINTAIN RELATIONSHIPS IN A WAY THAT MAKES IT IMPOSSIBLE TO RESOLVE PROBLEMS?**
● **ARE FAMILY MEMBERS TOO CLOSE (enmeshed) OR TOO DISTANT (disengaged)?**

YES →

NO

● Work with the family to help family members develop different and more appropriate responses, (e.g. stopping one person speaking for another, or challenging the claim that one person is not involved and it is not their problem).
● Allow the problem behaviour to occur then try to block the unhelpful behaviour and encourage other ways for them to react that are more likely to succeed.
  e.g. 'How did you decide that it would be best for your husband to explain your symptoms?'
  e.g. 'Will you tell me when he misses something out?'

IS THERE CONFUSION ABOUT WHO IS IN CONTROL?
e.g. are the children in control of their parents?

YES →

NO

● Challenge the assumption that an ineffective or non-existent executive function is acceptable for the family:
  e.g. 'How will you know when a decision needs to be made?"
  e.g. ' Who will think it's their job to make such a decision?'
● Do not allow yourself to agree that a problem is caused by one person (the 'scapegoat'). Try to create a description of the problem that shows the positive aspects of the behaviour being complained about.
  e.g. If someone asserts another family member has the problem, challenge this by saying 'Things are rarely as straight-forward as that, but tell me how you see the situation.'
  e.g. 'John has been keeping important information to himself. Why do you think he needs to overprotect you like that?'

ARE THE WAYS IN WHICH THE FAMILY TRIES TO SOLVE ITS PROBLEMS TOO RIGID OR CHAOTIC?

YES →

NO

● **If patterns are 'chaotic'**: help family to realise that such behaviour means no one can focus on sorting out the problem — comment on the way in which they talk and behave (i.e. the process), rather than lecture at them.
  e.g. 'Does what David just said help you to decide what to do about the children?'
  e.g. 'How can you help David be clearer about what he thinks should happen?'
● **If patterns are 'rigid'**: help the family not to keep repeating the same discussion — 'unbalance' things by introducing the unexpected to encourage new ways of functioning. Challenge: create more intensity (if you become more polite they will never be able to experiment).

● Check the family has been given relevant information about situation.
● Check whose problem it is.

IS IT THE PROFESSIONALS WHO HAVE THE PROBLEM?

NO

YES →

● Reassess and return to the beginning.

GO TO PART 3

If the family members think they will not cope in the future it is helpful to enable them to prioritise the worries since this breaks overwhelming worry into manageable parts. By looking at what has helped them so far, they can identify their strengths and resources. In this way they feel confirmed and can clarify problems, so that control is returned to them.

Is the family resisting making adjustments? If the family is not coping, members may accept advice on what to do. If the family is resisting such advice it is important to understand how the family and its individuals view things. It is quite common for a family to be having difficulty accepting the severity of the illness. Such denial may fluctuate from day to day, but when in denial the family will find it impossible to plan for the worst, leaving a strong residue of anxiety and fear. Patients can also be in the same situation, resulting in collusion, a 'conspiracy of silence'. See the flow diagram on *Breaking Bad News* for further information on denial and collusion. The family may be exhausted from the demands placed upon it and this exhaustion is often expressed by fixed attitudes and responses, with an inability to take in new information. Just asking how people have been coping will acknowledge their exhaustion and show that the team is sensitive to their difficulties.

Second order change

If the difficulties arising from the crisis are not solved by modifying the way they are being handled, second order changes may be needed.

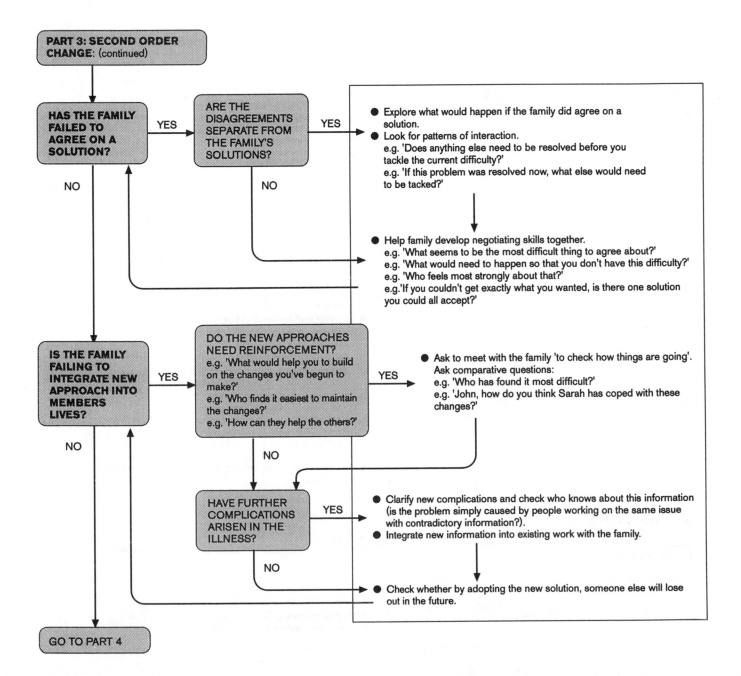

How does the family organise itself? The family's way of coping may be contributing to the problem, even if everyone has coped well before the present illness. The family needs the flexibility to change, but this will need the support of staff. It is difficult to suggest the need for change since this implies they have not coped in the past. In such circumstances it is important to acknowledge what has worked in the past:

'Up until now you've coped with everything life has thrown at you. But this time, you're saying things are not getting sorted, despite all your efforts. It doesn't look as if more of the same will make any difference. It looks like you need some new skills.'

Working with the family: Although it is often easy to see why things are not getting sorted out, it can be difficult to know how to ease the process. If you are helping the patient to say something important but upsetting, and the process is interrupted by the son with an unrelated question, it is important to challenge the way the son is contributing. Direct confrontation will only develop into silence or an argument, so it is better to ask a question about the process:

Professional: 'How did you decide that your son would need to protect all of you when difficult things were being said?'

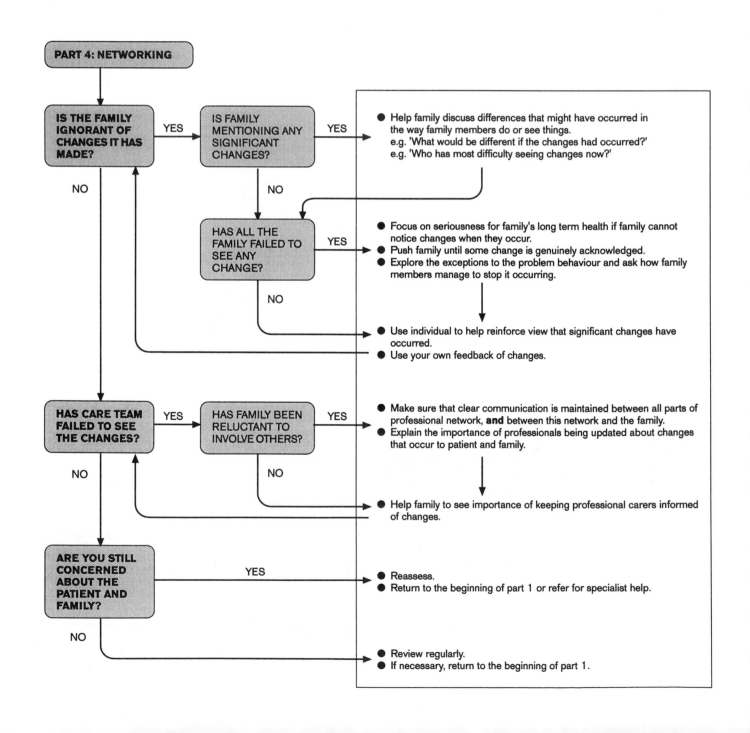

Mother: 'Well, we didn't.'

Professional: 'Oh, that's interesting. So how did he know if that's what you wanted?'

Mother: 'I don't know…I didn't want it. There are things I wanted to say to all of them.'

Professional: 'So how did your son get the impression that it was his job to help you in this way. Perhaps you could check that with him now.'

The other way to address unhelpful patterns of communication is to block communication with clear body language. This active type of intervention will only work when the family is confident in the professional, and it also requires some training, as it can generate anger.

Is there confusion about who is control? Families may find it difficult to make decisions because there is no agreement over who has the authority to make these decisions. By asking whether such a poor decision-making process is acceptable, you are challenging them to consider how they will know when a decision has been made.

It takes two or more to make a problem. The family may put off decisions and deny that anyone else is involved by creating a scapegoat:

'Dad has always been a worrier: he just won't discuss it with us. Can you sort him out?'

A helpful initial comment is:

'Things are rarely as straightforward as that, but tell me how *you* see the situation.'

This establishes that you do not agree with the assumption, but that there is still interest in hearing the family's views and experience. It is also helpful to describe the difficult behaviour in positive terms:

'You say that John is keeping important information to himself. Why do you think he needs to protect you like that?'

In this way the family is challenged with the notion of protection, but with the follow up that trying to be helpful does not always help.

Are the family solutions too rigid or too chaotic? It is natural for family members to retreat behind more rigid ways of coping, but if this fails to provide the control they are looking for, they will tend to react chaotically to the moment. The professional can help by supporting the family in regaining the 'middle ground' again, where they keep some useful patterns of behaviour but with some room for experimentation.

Is it the professionals who have the problem? This may happen for many reasons. For example, emotional identification with a patient can cloud the professional's judgement, increase patient dependence and may disrupt relationships between patient and family. We always need to look very carefully when we see a 'stuck and difficult' family to ensure that we are not in reality seeing reflected a 'stuck and difficult' team. In order to encourage a useful interaction between patient and team, it is helpful for individuals in the team to reflect on what they are doing with a patient and why. This will help in understanding what is happening in individual cases, as well as in furthering the professional development of the team member.

Has the family failed to agree on a solution? Failure to agree may be longstanding, in which case it is worth asking what would happen if they did agree on a solution? The disagreement may be helping them cope by avoiding the pain of what is happening; alternatively it may be clear that the old disagreement has to be resolved before going any further. The most difficult situation is when there is a longstanding disagreement the family does not wish to address, even though family members are desperate for a change to the present situation. In this situation it can be helpful to break down the problems to manageable parts.

Is the family failing to integrate change? Even when agreement has been reached about what to do next, and how to do it, it can still be difficult to maintain the changes. Reinforcement can help, such as meeting again in three weeks. The family may feel, however, that the situation is now different, believing that the old solutions no longer apply. This may be because of changes in the illness, in which case giving appropriate information allows all the family to work from the same information. With some families not all members are able to live with the solutions and this will require future work with the family.

Networking. Networking is concerned with effective communication within and between the professional team and the family.

Are the family or professionals unaware of how much they have done? There are many obstacles that prevent teams and families communicating and this can result in reluctance or failure to recognise the changes a family has made. Part of empowering them is helping them find acceptable ways of saying how they feel and what they need.

Are you still concerned?

If you feel uncertain about talking with a group of people, try sitting in on other people's interviews. Build up your confidence. You need to believe that starting the process of talking with families will not catapult you into uncharted and dangerous waters. Starting by clarifying the issues is immensely helpful to a group of people who are under great stress and are too caught up in the detail to be able to look at the wider picture. Use the skills of other members of the interdisciplinary team where necessary, and particularly when you feel more pro-active work needs to be done.

Acknowledgements

The authors would like to acknowledge the support and help of the following people in writing the original flow diagram: Catherine Adams, Judy Hildebrand, Hugh Jenkins, Len O'Connor, and Jürgen Schaufler.

Further Reading

Reference text

Doyle D, Hanks G and MacDonald N. eds. *Oxford Textbook of Medicine*. Oxford: Oxford University Press, 1993.

Palliative Care Journals

European Journal of Palliative Care. Chipping Norton: Hayward Medical Communications
(ISSN 1352–2779)

The Hospice Journal. New York: Haworth Press
(ISSN 0742–969X)

Journal of Pain and Symptom Management. New York: Elsevier
(ISSN 0885–3924)

The Journal of Palliative Care. Montreal: Clinical Research Institute of Montreal
(ISSN 0825-8597)

Palliative Medicine. London: Edward Arnold.
(ISSN 0269–2163)

Palliative care texts

Doyle D. *Caring for a Dying Relative*. Oxford: Oxford University Press, 1994.

Doyle D. *Domiciliary Palliative Care: A Guide to the Primary Care Team*. Oxford: Oxford University Press, 1994.

Regnard C and Tempest S. *A Guide to Symptom Relief in Advanced Cancer*, third edition. Manchester: Haigh and Hochland, 1992.

Saunders C, ed. *The Management of Terminal Malignant Disease*, third edition. London: Edward Arnold, 1993.

Stedeford A. *Facing Death: Patients, Families and Professionals*, second edition. Oxford: Sobell Publications, 1994.

Twycross RG and Lack SA. *Therapeutics in Terminal Cancer*, second edition. Edinburgh: Churchill Livingstone, 1990

Twycross RG and Lack SA. *Control of Alimentary Symptoms in Far Advanced Cancer*, 1986. Edinburgh: Churchill Livingstone.

Pain

Bonica JJ, ed. *The Management of Pain*, Volumes I and II, second edition. Philadelphia: Lea and Febiger, 1990.

Hanks GW and Justins DM. Cancer Pain: Management. *Lancet*, 1992; **339**: 1031–6.

Twycross RG. *Symptom Control in Far Advanced Cancer: Pain Relief*. second edition. London: Pitman, 1994.

Twycross RG. *Pain Relief in Advanced Cancer*. Edinburgh: Churchill Livingstone, 1994.

Tyrer SP. ed. *Psychology, Psychiatry and Chronic Pain*. Oxford: Butterworth Heineman, 1992.

Wall PD and Melzack R, eds, *Textbook of Pain*, third edition. Edinburgh: Churchill Livingstone, 1994.

Wells PE, Frampton V and Bowsher D, eds. *Pain: Management by Physiotherapy*. second edition. London: Butterworth Heinemann, 1994.

Dysphagia

Logemann JA. In: *Evaluation and Treatment of Swallowing Disorders*. San Diego: College Hill Press, 1983.

Regnard CFB. Dysphagia. In: Bates T ed. Palliation in Malignant Disease. Balliere's Clinical Oncology, 1987; **1**: 327–55.

Malignant ulcers

England F. Wound Management in Palliative Care. Contact: Palliative Care Nursing Group. RCN, 1993; Winter: 6–8.

Simms R and Fitzgerald V. *Management of Patients with Ulcerating/Fungating Malignant Breast Disease*. London: RCN Publication, 1985.

Grocott P. Practical Changes (Malignant Wounds). *Nursing Times*, 1993; **89**: 64–70.

Hastings D. Basic Care on Research (Fungating Lesions – Community). *Nursing Times*, 1993; **89**: 70–76.

Ivetic O and Lyne PA. Fungating and Ulcerating Lesions: a review of the literature. *J Adv Nurs*, 1990; **15**: 83–88.

Woodhouse P. Managing a Breast Wound. *Nursing Times* 1992; **88**: 72–75.

Confusion

Twycross RG and Lack SA. Neuropsychological Symptoms, In: *Therapeutics in Terminal Cancer*, second edition. Edinburgh: Churchill Livingstone, 1990: 81–99.

Twycross RG and Lack SA. Psychotropic Drugs, In: *Therapeutics in Terminal Cancer*, second edition. Edinburgh: Churchill Livingstone, 1990: 101–121.

The anxious person

Clark DM. Anxiety states – panic in generalised anxiety. In: Hawton K, Salkvovskis EM, Kirk J and Clark DM, eds. *Cognitive Behaviour Therapy for Psychiatric Problems: a Practical Guide*. New York: Oxford Medical Publications, 1989. pp. 52–96.

Moorey S and Greer S. *Psychological Therapy for Patients with Cancer: A New Approach*. Oxford: Heinemann, 1989.

Breaking bad news

Buckman R. *How to Break Bad News: A Guide for Health Care Professionals*. London: Papermac, 1992.

Handling difficult questions

Faulkner A and Maguire P. *Talking to Cancer Patients and their Relatives*. Oxford: Oxford University Press, 1994.

Index